MW00748316

THE LIFE AND DESTRUCTION
OF SAINT MARY'S HOSPITAL

THE LIFE AND DESTRUCTION OF SAINT MARY'S HOSPITAL

Jaimie McEvoy

with a foreword by Dr. Irwin F. Stewart

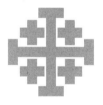

SAINT MARY'S HEALTH FOUNDATION

Copyright © 2008 Saint Mary's Health Foundation

All rights reserved.
Printed in Canada.

Dust jacket: *Front, top,* Saint Mary's Hospital, c. 1957, courtesy New Westminster Museum and Archives. *Bottom,* demolition of Saint Mary's Hospital, 2005, courtesy Jaimie McEvoy. *Back, left to right,* Saint Mary's Hospital, 1887, courtesy New Westminster Museum and Archives, manuscript #302; nurse Ann Jackson and Native child, Saint Mary's Hospital, 1918, courtesy Saint Paul's Hospital Archives; A view of Saint Mary's Hospital after years of development, courtesy New Westminster Museum and Archives.

This book is published by Saint Mary's Health Foundation (formerly Saint Mary's Hospital Foundation) in memory of Saint Mary's Hospital. The Foundation provides support for health care through grants to hospitals and other health-care providers. Proceeds from the sale of this book will be used for this purpose.

Donations may also be made to:
        Saint Mary's Health Foundation of New Westminster
        Box 16033, 617 Belmont Street
        New Westminster, BC V3M 6W6

Library and Archives Canada Cataloguing in Publication

McEvoy, Jaimie, 1965–
    The life and destruction of Saint Mary's Hospital / Jaimie McEvoy.

ISBN 978-0-9811365-0-9

    1. Saint Mary's Hospital (New Westminster, B.C.)—History. 2. Medical care—British Columbia—New Westminster—History. 3. New Westminster (B.C.) —History. I. Saint Mary's Health Foundation II. Title.
RA983.N482S34 2008   362.1109711'33   C2008-907487-4

Nov. 23, 2016

To Jackie Jacob
Congratulations on
the BCIT nursing
programme.

This book is dedicated to Saint Mary's Hospital, the
thousands of patients who found comfort there, its
caring staff, volunteers and supporters who defended
the hospital to the end.

Bill Walsh
Director
SMH. F.

Contents

Foreword

THIS BOOK TELLS THE STORY OF SAINT MARY'S HOSPITAL in New Westminster, British Columbia, from its founding in 1887 by the Sisters of Charity of Providence through to its demolition in 2005. It is not possible, however, to relate Saint Mary's history without telling the story of health care in British Columbia and New Westminster over the past 150 years. In the beginning, the province's health care was chaotic, with care dispensed by inexperienced ships' doctors and outright quacks and charlatans, jails crowded with the mentally ill, and epidemics that decimated the white and First Nations populations. This period includes the creation of this province in the young Dominion of Canada, the Klondike Gold Rush, two world wars, smallpox, cholera and influenza epidemics, the Great Fire of New Westminster, numerous health-care reforms and the ultimate betrayal that closed Saint Mary's doors forever after 117 years of faithful and compassionate service.

Administrative jealousy and political expediency conspired to close Saint Mary's in 2003, despite the protests of thousands of British Columbians who attempted to keep the hospital open, having recognized that Saint Mary's had become one of the finest surgical centres in the province. Many people are still confused and angry over the intrigue and political manoeuvrings that closed their community hospital forever. Sadly, since taking office in 2001, the Liberal Government led by Premier Gordon Campbell has closed a number of community hospitals in British Columbia and cut back numerous other health services. The closure of these facilities has had a severe impact on the health of British Columbians, particularly at a time when the health-care system in the province is unable to cope with the needs of an expanding and aging population. Now it is clear to most that health care in British Columbia is in chaos and the provincial government has not found a prescription to make it better. Wait-lists for treatment of almost every kind, but particularly surgery, continue to get longer. We're told that some surgical wait-lists are improving. But how can we know? There isn't a good reliable "master wait-list" for us to check. Emergency departments in many hospitals are unable to cope with increasing volume and hundreds of needed hospital beds lie empty because of inadequate staffing levels and financial resources.

The Fraser Health Authority announced on June 28, 2006, a $228-million package to upgrade Surrey Memorial Hospital, including a $126-million outpatient care centre that will be built and operational by 2009. But the outpatient care centre already existed at Saint Mary's Hospital as well as a 100-bed in-patient acute and geriatric service, but all of this was sold for a meagre $4.1 million.

Health care in our province has gone from chaos in 1887 to chaos in 2008.

—DR. IRWIN F. STEWART, C.M., B.A., M.D., F.R.C.S.

CHIEF OF STAFF, SAINT MARY'S HOSPITAL, 1976–1981

1

The Need for Compassionate Health Care
1858–1863

"My father was so opposed to vaccination for any purpose that he slept with a revolver under his pillow when the authorities were forcibly vaccinating people."

—EUNICE HARRISON[1]

EUNICE HARRISON WAS A CHILD OF FIVE when the 1862–63 smallpox epidemic hit New Westminster and she became deathly sick. Doctor A.W.S. Black confirmed her illness as smallpox and immediately quarantined the house and all inside. Eunice would later recall being thickly wrapped like a mummy and sleeping between her parents as they tried to keep her warm during her sickness, and she remembered having her hands tied behind her back to prevent the scratching that can leave smallpox scars. Miraculously, her parents, as well as another couple and their two children who were guests in the Harrison home and also quarantined, never became ill.

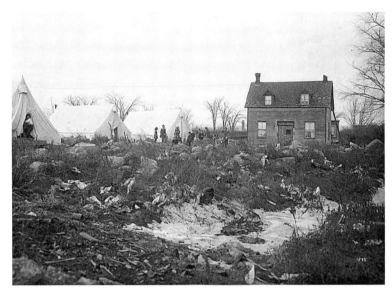

Smallpox tents on a quarantine island circa 1875. The quarantine hospital built in 1899 on New Westminster's Poplar Island would have been similar.
PHOTOGRAPH BY WILLIAM JAMES TOPLEY, LIBRARY AND ARCHIVES CANADA, PA-009184.

Smallpox was an ongoing concern in the Pacific Northwest in the nineteenth century, with the first of these devastating epidemics occurring in 1836–38. The 1862–63 outbreak began in Victoria after the arrival of an infected sailor from San Francisco. When it spread to First Nations groups camped on the outskirts of the city, the authorities burned their camps and drove them away. As they travelled home they carried the disease with them, spreading it to the mainland.

Victims of the disease would feel a sudden fever, a strong headache and a tremendous pain in the back followed by red spots that soon became blisters and then open pustules. Although a vaccine had been developed as early as 1796, it tended to be distributed only after the disease had already broken out.

It was also difficult to convince many people, Native and non-Native, to be vaccinated because they saw it as an injection of the disease. Many were so opposed that, like Eunice Harrison's father, they were prepared to shoot anyone who attempted to vaccinate them or any member of their families. "Father," Eunice wrote in her diary, "said that no one was going to force him against his will."[2]

There were some heroic efforts to save lives, however. Doctor John Helmcken vaccinated several hundred people in the Victoria area. A Hudson's Bay Company post trader in the Shuswap area vaccinated local Natives. The Reverend John Sheepshanks, the first priest of New Westminster's Holy Trinity Anglican Church, travelled to Williams Lake, vaccinating every Native person he could along the way, and in 1862 alone Father Leon Fouquet of the Oblates of Mary Immaculate (OMI) made at least thirty-five trips to vaccinate the people living in forty Native "rancheries"—small villages—against smallpox. Oblate records show that he vaccinated some 8,000 people, saving thousands of lives in the process.

In those trying times it was difficult to obtain professional health care on the mainland of British Columbia. The only hospital was maintained solely for the men of the Columbia Detachment of the Royal Engineers, commonly known as the "Sappers." In 1858 the British government had sent the Engineers under the command of Colonel Richard Clement Moody to survey the new crown colony of British Columbia and build a capital city at New Westminster. Among the more than two hundred engineers and their families who embarked for the new colony was Staff Assistant-Surgeon John Vernon Seddall, who was expected to keep the troops fit and healthy. He had begun this task while still aboard the *Thames City* en route to British Columbia from Gravesend by ordering all his charges to drink lime juice, the standard Royal Navy scurvy preventive, thus earning himself a reputation as an effective practitioner. (The trip was not a happy one for Seddall as his fine, waist-length, reddish-brown beard was smeared by the tar and pitch on the ship, forcing him to shave it off.) As a qualified military doctor, Seddall would have had "a diploma from the College of Physicians and Surgeons. To qualify for such a diploma he would have spent six years attending various courses covering such subjects as anatomy and dissection, surgery, medicine, chemistry, midwifery, and the preparation of drugs. In addition to this (apart from the fact that he had to be between twenty-one and twenty-five years old and single as well) an army surgeon had to have eighteen months experience and be able to provide recommendations from responsible people."[3]

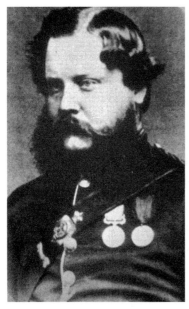

Seddall's small "Sappers Hospital," built in 1859, was noteworthy for its "Spartan simplicity,"[4] but it was well equipped, and Seddall had the assistance of hospital orderly Henry Hazel, who can

Staff Assistant-Surgeon John Vernon Seddall, New Westminster's first doctor, arrived with the Royal Engineers to build the city as the new colonial capital of British Columbia. PHOTOGRAPH COURTESY OF NEW WESTMINSTER PUBLIC LIBRARY #996.

reasonably be described as the mainland's first nurse. However, this hospital was strictly for the use of army patients recovering from surgery, exceptions being made for non-military persons only in the case of true emergencies. But Dr. Seddall remained in the colony for just five years; he was one of the Royal Engineers who chose not to stay behind in British Columbia when the detachment's work was done in building the new colony. He returned to England on November 14, 1863.

In those days, the only other option available to non-military residents of the mainland for hospital care was to travel to the Royal Hospital in Victoria, the capital of the crown colony of Vancouver Island. It had not been the first hospital established on the Island. At the outbreak of the Crimean War in 1854, a contingent of the Royal Navy had been moved north from Chile to Esquimalt in case the war spread to the Pacific, and the Navy had built three small hospital huts there the following year to accommodate possible casualties. Fortunately, that eventuality never arose so the huts were never put to use. Then in 1858, after a desperately ill man was abandoned on the Reverend Edward Cridge's doorstep, the Reverend, Dr. John Helmcken and others had converted a vacant cottage in Victoria into a public hospital. A year later the Royal Hospital was founded there.

The Royal charged patients directly for treatment, but the government also levied a one-dollar tax on both island and mainland residents to support the hospital. This charge was, of course, resented by the people of the mainland, given the difficulty of transporting the sick or injured across the Strait of Georgia. When in 1862 the colonial government proposed doubling the tax, New Westminster residents, faced with a distant government that believed there need be only one hospital to serve both Pacific-coast colonies, tried to convince authorities to move the hospital from Victoria to their capital, arguing that the sea breezes in Victoria were bad for patients' recovery. Their argument fell on deaf ears.

A few doctors practised in New Westminster at this time but not much is known about them. Miners in the Interior tended to have better access to medicine as doctors often followed them to their camps, knowing that these men could usually afford to pay and that the hazards of mining would generate a lot of business. None of these doctors, though, worked in any kind of a hospital and one can only speculate on where and how any needed surgery was conducted. Some of them might have had formal training, but often this was not the case. Most patients tended to be suspicious of the training of their doctors anyway, especially since in the young colony no process existed to register or check the credentials of any of them. As well, British immigrants tended to see Canadian-trained doctors as second rate, though many more were suspicious of American doctors because standards varied so much from state to state. One doctor in Victoria inspired patients' mistrust by falling down almost constantly. His explanation for this was that the government had employed a Chinese man to follow him around and throw invisible projectiles at the back of his neck. A local reverend speculated that whisky likely had more to do with the doctor's unsteadiness on his feet than any government conspiracy involving Chinese men and invisible missiles.

Even trained doctors often treated conditions for which there was not really any cure. In Yale in 1861 a British-trained doctor named Max Fifer was shot dead by his patient Robert

Wall who was upset that the doctor's medicines were not curing him of his impotence. He blamed Fifer for his permanent dizziness, but Wall likely had syphilis and none of the doctor's treatments could have cured him. However, like many doctors at that time, Fifer was probably just trying to make a living in a completely free-for-all system, willing to have his patients pay while he tried to do something for them when, in reality, he could do nothing. Other medical practitioners, such as Dr. Crain whose office was on Columbia Street in New Westminster, supplemented the meagre income from their practices by selling perfumes, soap and other personal body products. When in 1867 all doctors were required to produce credentials, register and be licensed, some of those who were practising medicine suddenly quit the colony. However, even then, these new requirements were not always enforced, and it was not until 1886 when a College of Physicians and Surgeons was established in British Columbia that the law became effective.

Up to the middle of the nineteenth century nursing was not considered a reputable profession for women. During wars the care of wounded soldiers was undertaken by the prostitutes who followed the armies; in hospitals on the homefront, since most of the patients were injured working men, men were hired to nurse them. Female nurses were relegated to tending patients in their homes where they often doubled as maids. This situation only began to change in the latter half of the nineteenth century as the result of the publicity garnered by Florence Nightingale's group of nurses ministering to British soldiers during the Crimean War (1853–1856) and by her treatise, *Notes on Nursing*, published in 1860.

As a result of the difficulty in getting medical help, many

people just tried to survive disease and injury without medical care. Some used cure-all potions like the well-advertised Holloway's Pills and Ointments. The pills were supposedly imbued with a magic power to cure almost everything from female irregularity to venereal diseases, indigestion and tumours. The ointments promised to cure insect bites as well as cancer. There were also potions such as Foo Choo's Balsam of Shark's Oil, advertised as a miracle cure for deafness. And if the disease didn't kill the patient, the medicine might: a man named Alfred Clayton, who suffered from insomnia, died of the cure in January 1884 when he overdosed on the laudanum prescribed to help him sleep.

There was no accommodation for the mentally ill in the early days of British Columbia, although as a result of the rainy climate and isolation, many of the Hudson's Bay employees are reported to have suffered from depression. One man, in fact, became so depressed that his wife and children had to take over his duties, and in Fort Victoria in 1850, another young man, after a period of irrational behaviour, suddenly attacked the Hudson's Bay Company's surgeon, John Helmcken. The young man was incarcerated in the company's jail where he was diagnosed as insane, presumably by the same Dr. Helmcken. He was then put on board a Hudson's Bay ship and sent back to England. This same process was followed for future cases of mental breakdown, making the establishment of any kind of care facility for the mentally ill in this remote little colony unnecessary.

When gold was discovered on the Fraser River in 1858, it seemed to the British subjects already resident here that an unusual number of the American gold seekers coming north from the California goldfields were "lunatics." Rumours then began to spread that California's officials had taken advantage of the mass northward movement to release people from their asylums and prisons. Thus, it seemed reasonable to officials here to ship them back, and for a while all those American gold seekers who were deemed to be lunatics were sent back to such places as California's Napa Asylum. Soon, however, the government of California began to insist that many of these people were not Americans, and they would accept no more unless the British government paid for their care. This did not happen, and the jails in both Victoria and New Westminster were then used to house them.

Most of the early Hudson's Bay employees and the colonists and miners who came after them experienced some degree of mental and emotional turmoil in leaving their densely populated homelands and even greater distress when they faced the vastness of this distant wilderness. Thus, when an uncommonly high proportion of miners seemed to be suffering from mental illness, it was gradually recognized that it was the result of the excitement of the gold rush combined with the many disappointed hopes and the effects of isolation. Pioneer women, cooped up with their children in remote and inadequate log cabins during the long dismal BC winters, were especially prone to depression. On November 4, 1859, the *British Colonist* newspaper reported that:

> Mrs. Crote, wife of one of the sappers and miners had been in a desponding way for some time . . . When the news about the murder of three men by Indians at the mouth of the river reached her, it turned her brain completely and

she was heard to say that sooner than the Indians should kill her children she would kill them herself.[5]

Mrs. Crote did kill herself and two of her children. The jury deemed that she was temporarily insane, which at that time was seen as a fact of life that one could really do nothing about.

In 1861 New Westminster's municipal council began its long tradition of being directly involved in health-care matters and formed a committee to investigate the need for a hospital. The committee discovered that there were a number of sick and injured men in the city who were in serious condition without money or someone to care for them and, as a consequence, would die or become permanently disabled. As a result, the council decided that the community would have to raise funds to care for the destitute and seriously injured. About this time Father Leon Fouquet, OMI, who recognized the desperate need for a hospital on the mainland, simply announced that he would go ahead and open a Catholic hospital. His statement, which was well publicized, galvanized the largely Anglican town establishment into action and, within a month of Fouquet's declaration, two

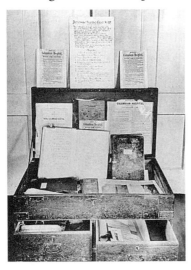

The medical chest of the Royal Engineers. Two chests like this one served as the entire medical inventory of mainland British Columbia in 1858. PHOTOGRAPHER UNKNOWN, ARTIFACTS PICTURED LOCATED AT NEW WESTMINSTER MUSEUM AND ARCHIVES.

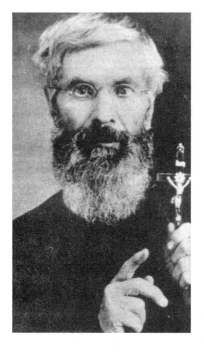

Father Leon Fouquet, who in 1861 announced plans to found a Catholic hospital in response to the colonial government's failure to open a hospital on the mainland of British Columbia. PHOTOGRAPH COURTESY OF MISSION COMMUNITY ARCHIVES.

public meetings had been held to organize a town hospital. Perhaps the priest's announcement had hit a nerve in the long-suffering mainland populace. Colonel Moody, who with his Royal Engineers was the founder and builder of New Westminster, became the first president of the board of management of the Royal Columbian Hospital.

However, the following spring, when smallpox began raging across Vancouver Island, the people of New Westminster faced the fact that they still had no facility to cope with an epidemic. That summer the first two victims in the city were local Natives, the third a white resident from the neglected west end of town, but the disease soon spread rapidly into the more respectable parts of the city. As a result of this crisis, the Royal Columbian Hospital was opened in October of that same year, not at its present location in Sapperton, but at Agnes and Clement (now Fourth) streets in downtown New Westminster. The central part of the new hospital building housed the surgery and the steward's quarters, with wards constructed to either

side. Though most of the hospital was made of wood, the walls
between the surgery and the two wards were brick so the patients in the wards would not be disturbed by the sounds coming from the surgery. Anaesthetics existed but they were often
inadequate or simply not used as some doctors actually believed
that screaming was good for the patient and would help reduce
pain. When the Columbia Detachment of the Royal Engineers
was disbanded a year after the Royal Columbian was built, the
new hospital fell heir to all of its predecessor's supplies, including the furniture, bedding, Dr. Seddall's instruments and supplies, and even the large and at that time very valuable bath,
complete with all its pipes and fittings.

Only seven patients were admitted when the hospital
opened because the northeast wing had been reserved to host a
ball to celebrate the opening as well as the twenty-first birthday
of the Prince of Wales, later Edward VII. Sixty men who were

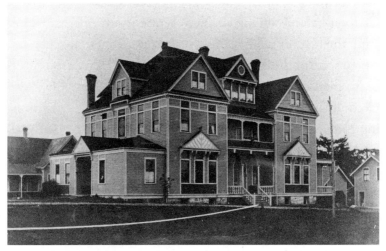

Royal Columbian Hospital as it appeared circa 1903. PHOTOGRAPH COURTESY OF
NEW WESTMINSTER PUBLIC LIBRARY #1058.

considered New Westminster's leading citizens held a dinner where they made speeches and many toasts. Their womenfolk were fetched only when it was time to dance.

By February 1863 the new hospital was already badly in debt. Most of the patients were unable to pay the required $10 per week, and it quickly became clear that raising money to build a hospital was an entirely different matter from continually raising money to keep it going. A main source of revenue now came from concerts organized by former Royal Engineers who had several good musicians and singers within their ranks. It was not until 1865 that the colonial government began to provide greater financial assistance, but in return the government required two of its own to be appointed to the seven-man board. That year, despite there still being some debt, Dr. McNaughton Jones and Dr. A.W.S. Black, the hospital's two medical officers, were paid for the first time. Doctor Black, an Australian, had practised in the goldfields of California and the Cariboo before coming to New Westminster.[6] Richard Holland, the first hospital steward, was paid $75 per month.

In spite of the establishment of a hospital, universal access to hospital care had not yet been achieved because the Royal Columbian had specific restrictions that prevented its meeting the needs of many in the community. To begin with, all admissions required the approval of both the hospital's chief medical officer and a local magistrate. Except when children required emergency treatment for serious injuries—broken bones or burns from house fires—families were expected to care for their own children. And, perhaps the worst restriction of all, the hospital would only accept patients who were considered curable, eliminating any kind of treatment for people whose condition would likely lead to death. It is hard to believe today, but for decades the policy was that the more likely a patient was to die the less likely he was to be eligible for admission. Hospitals were, therefore, not so much about the care of the ill and injured as they were about emergency treatment and surgery.

All surgery at this time posed a threat to life and limb—in fact, surgery to remove a limb was the most common type of operation. Rather than risk gangrene, the surgeon would simply amputate an arm or leg with a bad compound fracture. However, because conditions in many hospitals were not sterile, patients often died from infection after surgery. Bullet and knife wounds were also not uncommon in those early days, though most patients were admitted for disease. There also seemed to be an epidemic of paralysis, sometimes requiring several years of hospitalization; this was generally the result of late-stage syphilis, which was very prevalent among a population made up largely of single young men. Sadly, suicide also seems to have been a fairly common response to serious illness or injury, particularly among the many labouring men of the colony, who chose it as the best alternative to a long and painful death or desperate poverty with nowhere to go if they were no longer able to work.

Women were very rarely hospitalized as men did most of the dangerous work that resulted in injuries and, unlike men, they were rarely involved in accidents and injuries caused by drunkenness or fighting. Women almost always gave birth at home. The first doctor in New Westminster, Dr. Seddall, was required as part of his training to take courses in midwifery, but for the most part doctors were never present at births at all as women actually tried to avoid involving them. A doctor was generally sent for only when something went wrong.

Tragically, the new Royal Columbian Hospital also refused to admit mentally ill persons. Instead, sending "lunatics" back to their country of origin was still seen as the most desirable option, though it could be expensive, and the settler population and gold miners did not have the Hudson's Bay Company to foot the bill. Sometimes, if the subject was deemed worthy and had not fallen into insanity through some sinful behaviour, the public would raise the necessary money through donations. So it was that a Mr. Templeton was sent home in 1863 after the sum of $59 had been raised for his food, transportation and the services of a keeper to act as an escort. This incident caused the self-named Amor de Cosmos (Lover of the Universe), founder of the *British Colonist* newspaper and later premier of British Columbia, to wonder in print whether it would not be better to establish a local lunatic asylum. But in the end the practice of deporting the mentally ill only ceased when it became too expensive.

At this period in New Westminster's history the mentally ill were usually left to fend for themselves unless considered violent or dangerous, in which case they were held in the jail. In fact, the New Westminster jail on Clarkson Street in the downtown district served as the asylum for the entire mainland, and the screaming that came from within it was a source of much complaint from the neighbours. Many of the "lunatics" held in its five-foot by seven-foot cells were actually in the latter stages of other diseases and most died within a year of incarceration. However, at times the cells were too full of the mentally ill to house any actual lawbreakers, and offenders had to be chained up in the jail's kitchen or even out in the woodshed.

The conditions in the jail became so deplorable that in August 1861 Judge Begbie appointed a grand jury to investigate it. They found a Native man in one cell dying of tuberculosis, kept there simply because there was nowhere else for him to go. The poor man had become skeletal, his bed a straw pallet on the floor. Also incarcerated were two violent, mentally ill men who were kept in straitjackets and irons. Everything had been removed from their cells, including bedding, to prevent its destruction. They slept on the bare floor and were left in their own filth. One of them usually destroyed any clothing he was given and so had been left nude since the previous February; he died a few weeks later. Captain C.J. Pritchard, the lone warder who lived with his wife in the jail until his death in 1870, was generally seen as a kind and compassionate man. He maintained the premises in good condition and did the best he could to give care to the ill and tolerate the screams of the insane.

Even after the Royal Columbian Hospital was founded in 1862, those who were mentally ill were still housed in the jail because the hospital had no mandate or interest in taking them into an institution that was so limited in staff and capacity. In 1863 after a mentally ill man had somehow been admitted, the hospital board wrote to jail warden Chartres Brew to demand his removal:

Sir,

I am directed by the Board of Management of this hospital to request that you kindly cause the removal of an insane man at present here. His presence, so near the other patients, is attended not only with inconvenience, but with serious danger; his shouts and ravings retarding greatly the recovery of other inmates. You will not, they are sure, fail to recognize . . . that the hospital was never intended to be other than an institution for the curable sick; and that to appropriate its fund for the maintenance of a lunatic, whose condition of insanity is likely to be lasting, would be wrong. At some future day the Government may think fit to propose a special grant to this hospital, on account of the lunatics in the Colony, then of course . . . various arrangements could be made that are not practicable now.[7]

While the public had been appalled in 1861 when they learned of the terrible conditions in the jail, another jury investigating conditions in 1870 noted that none of the recommendations of the previous report had been implemented and that obviously ill patients were still kept there because they were either not eligible or too poor for entrance into a hospital.

It was not until negotiations were complete for BC to become a province of Canada that it was realized that an asylum would not be part of the confederation package provided by the Dominion. Therefore, in 1872 the provincial government finally opened one in Victoria's old Royal Hospital, and for a few years after that all patients diagnosed with mental illnesses on the British Columbia mainland were shipped over to Vancouver Island. But the institution was poorly run by E.A. Sharpe, who confounded staff when, as his first act, he ordered two hundred pounds of butter though the facility had no means to refrigerate it. Subsequent investigations revealed abuse of staff, mismanagement and stress among patients as Sharpe regulated their lives at a whim.

The provincial government then began to explore the idea of creating an asylum in New Westminster to satisfy officials in that city who were demanding that at least some of the province's public facilities should be established in the city that had once been the capital of the mainland colony. A letter was sent from Victoria to New Westminster's Dr. A.W.S. Black asking if any of the old buildings left behind by the sappers might be used. Doctor Black wholeheartedly supported their use for this purpose and reported that the cost of renovating them would be $700 to $900. Unfortunately, though the buildings were intact and well located and had a good water supply, converting them into an asylum never went forward. Thus, a year later when a local man began urging others to rally behind him to attack the United States and he was deemed clearly insane, the authorities, having discovered there was no room for him in the Victoria asylum, made the usual arrangements to incarcerate him in a local jail cell.

In 1878 New Westminster finally won its campaign to have an insane asylum, but the new institution had problems from the start. Two superintendents of construction were fired at the outset because they had taken considerable shortcuts in both the construction and the quality of the materials, and the work was still ongoing when the legislature in Victoria decided that, ready or not, the new institution would accept patients. During the debate, the notorious Mr. Smith said words to the effect that he had always regarded New Westminster as the proper place for lunatics, and a certain Dr. Ash declared that it didn't matter that the place was poorly built and incomplete because it should not be too comfortable anyway in order to prevent fakers from moving in. And so on May 17, 1878, twelve male and four female patients were sent from Victoria to the unfinished and wholly unsuitable buildings, accompanied by staff including the legendary Flora Ross.

In less than a year, the facility, built to accommodate twenty-eight patients, already housed forty-one. Within a few months Dr. McNaughton Jones resigned as the resident physician and was replaced by Dr. Thomas Robert McInnes, an American who had been a doctor on the Confederate side in the American Civil War and who would later become mayor of New Westminster and then Lieutenant-Governor of British Columbia. Although McInnes attended mainly to his private practice and only visited the institution every few days, he had

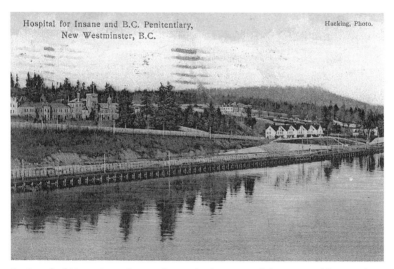

Hospital for Insane and B.C. Penitentiary, New Westminster, B.C.

Hacking, Photo.

Postcard of New Westminster shows the location of the original hospital at the BC Penitentiary, with the Provincial Hospital for the Insane property to the left. JAIMIE MCEVOY PRIVATE COLLECTION.

a serious drinking problem and was often absent for days or even weeks at a time. In 1879 the official death rate among patients there was about 30 percent, but many of the deaths were simply left unreported, and this state of affairs persisted in various ways at the institution for many years. By 1881 the building was literally falling apart, its chimney had collapsed, and there was a break in the Glen Brook dam that supplied its water.

Unfortunately, the scandals continued at the asylum, and the institution became known as either a place of compassionate refuge or a place of abuse, depending on the time period and the particular staff in that part of the institution. An 1892 investigation of a patient suicide found that the man had died while in restraints and locked in a closet. The investigators found that in the men's ward the patients were forced to wear white drill uniforms with a little star to mark them as mental patients. In the basement they discovered a cage that had been used to forcibly duck violent male patients completely into cold water, a practice that was quite literally right out of the Dark Ages. In contrast, Flora Ross had decorated the women's ward like a normal home, including plants and a piano, and she had instituted ball games. She also kept impeccable records of any use of restraint and punishment. Despite this, no one seems to have thought that this very experienced and capable woman should head the whole institution.

2

Building Saint Mary's Hospital
1866–1887

AS THE CARIBOO GOLD RUSH began winding down in 1866, the two British colonies of Vancouver Island and British Columbia sank into an economic recession. This prompted officials in London to decide that administration costs could be cut by combining the two colonies, and unfortunately, it was Victoria, not New Westminster, that was chosen as the capital of the combined colony. Thus, businesses fled to the Island capital, and the mainland city sank deeper into recession.

Then to add to the city's woes, in the summer of 1868 smallpox broke out among the shacks at the Native rancherie at the foot of New Westminster's Tenth Street near the Fraser River. The authorities reacted by burning all the dwellings, effectively destroying one of New Westminster's oldest established aboriginal communities. After the epidemic was over, they also burned the four-bed smallpox hospital, and the Royal Columbian Hospital board finally vaccinated the remaining local Native people against smallpox. (When a smallpox epidemic occurred again in 1879, whites were cared for in hospital and non-whites were quarantined in a building on McBride Boulevard and also possibly in a small building on Poplar Island.)

As the recession continued, some doctors left town, leaving Dr. A.W. S. Black, who remained the medical officer at the Royal Columbian Hospital, as the city's only doctor, but in 1871 he was found dead on the road between New Westminster and Burrard Inlet, having apparently been thrown from his horse.[8] The hospital had difficulty finding someone to replace him, someone willing to take on the combined job of working for the hospital and the jail, while still running a private practice to make a living. A certain Dr. Thornber applied and served for a while but was fired that same year when he could not produce credentials proving he actually was a doctor.

Meanwhile, Father Leon Fouquet, whose plan to provide New Westminster with a Catholic hospital had been forestalled by the construction of the Royal Columbian Hospital in 1862, had built a small hospital for Native people near Saint Charles Church in New Westminster[9] before transferring his attention farther up the Fraser River to found Saint Mary's Mission to minister to the Native population there. Even without Fouquet's leadership, however, the Catholic community of New Westminster had put their wholehearted support behind the new Royal Columbian Hospital. In fact, in the early 1880s James Morrison and W.H. Keary, the president and secretary of the hospital board, wrote to the local newspapers, openly criticizing the city's other denominations after only the Episcopalian and Catholic churches had responded to a request for extra collection plates to support the local hospital. But, in spite of these efforts, disease, fires and industrial accidents continued to test the ability of the hospital's limited facilities and its small medical staff to cope.

The truth was that British Columbia—which had become a province of Canada in July 1871—suffered from too few hospitals, charlatan doctors and discrimination in health care. Syphilis was endemic and everywhere on the streets of the cities men could be seen with the shuffling gait adopted by sufferers of the disease. Tuberculosis was common and effective treatment was non-existent; until the bacillus was isolated in 1890, the notion that this disease was caused by little creatures was largely seen as the stuff of lunatic minds. Cases of leprosy cropped up from time to time, and in 1882 a Chinese man was lynched in New Westminster by his compatriots when it was found that he had the disease. It wasn't until 1891 that the government reacted by establishing a leper colony on D'Arcy Island.

Most of these diseases were especially rampant among the poor, a fact that did eventually come to concern the wealthier people in the city, though only after the devastating 1891 typhoid epidemic. In 1886, the year before Saint Mary's Hospital opened, a man was found dying of typhoid on the streets of Vancouver. There was neither hospital nor doctor to send him to, so the coroner was called instead, even though the man was still alive. As nearly always happened with victims of diseases like smallpox and typhoid fever, this man had been evicted from his hotel, forcing him to contend with the ravages of typhoid alone on the street. Those who owned houses might be quarantined in their homes, but no hotelier wanted to house the ill and risk having his entire business closed down. For the poor, as well, there was no access to a hospital or a doctor, and they simply coped with their injuries and illnesses as best they could. They continued to die of exposure and starvation; some simply froze to death.

However, back in 1864, Father Louis-Joseph d'Herbomez, a member of the Oblates of Mary Immaculate, had become vicar apostolic for the Catholic Church of British Columbia and had established his base in New Westminster. Recognizing the formidable size of the province's problems, he became determined to see the establishment of new Catholic schools, orphanages and hospitals. In the opinion of d'Herbomez, despite the generosity of British Columbians, the needs of the local sick and the poor had simply not been met and were not likely to be met without intervention. "In civilized countries, there are always well-to-do and charitable persons who are happy to open hospitals and support them financially. In a new country such as ours, where people are just beginning to be established, we cannot expect such generosity. However, each one willingly donates, sometimes even from his own need. Where orphans and the sick are concerned, one cannot depend entirely on public generosity, and then one must find other resources. . . . Hospitals and orphanages are indispensable."[10]

Although d'Herbomez knew that the existing missions in the Pacific Northwest were already short of the support they needed, on October 30, 1875, he wrote to Sister Praxedes of the Sisters of Charity of the House of Providence (generally known as the Sisters of Providence) in Oregon to invite them to tour British Columbia in the hope that they would establish a mission here. "As you see," he wrote, "the harvest is great, but the labourers are too few, it is distressing! This is why I appeal to your congregation, whose zeal and dedication are so well known to us."[11] Then, in his determination to persuade the Sisters to assist, he assured them of the support of both Catholics and non-Catholics. "You are awaited with such anticipation, not only by the Catholics but also by our separated brethren, who wish for nothing better than the opportunity to help you in your charitable works, such as hospitals and orphanages."[12]

Although the Sisters apparently did make a tour of the new Canadian province, no new Sisters of Providence mission was undertaken there at that time. But things finally began to happen in 1886. In the spring of that year the regional governing body of the Sisters of Providence in Vancouver, Washington

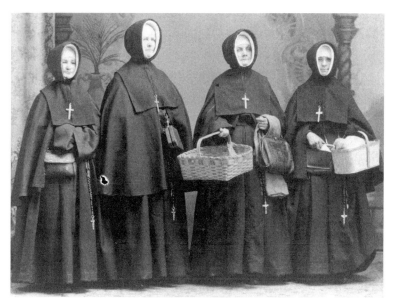

The Sisters of Providence travelled widely to visit the sick and the poor in their homes. NEW WESTMINSTER MUSEUM AND ARCHIVES MANUSCRIPT #302.

Territory, at last began debating the feasibility of building a hospital in New Westminster because they had recently been joined by four new Canadian Sisters from the Mother House in Montreal. They were, however, already committed to building a hospital in Spokane, and Mother Amable in Montreal questioned the wisdom of beginning two in the same year. "How you can handle two buildings at the same time and at such a distance apart, I do not know,"[13] she wrote. But the Sisters were not deterred. The record of their deliberations advises that:

> On the fifteenth day of June, eighteen hundred and eighty six at a meeting of the Corporation of the Sisters of Charity of the House of Providence, Vancouver, W.T. [Washington Territory], it was agreed to build an hospital in the city of New Westminster, B.C.
>
> Sister Joseph of the S.H. [Sacred Heart], Treasurer.
> Sister John of the Cross, Pres.[14]

On July 4, Sister Joseph and another Sister arrived in New Westminster from Vancouver, Washington Territory, to buy land and arrange for a contractor to build the hospital. Two days later they were joined by two more Sisters, and the four of them began a begging tour of the city to raise money toward construction; within days they had $3,000. By July 9 they were already back in Washington Territory where they formalized the decisions made in New Westminster:

> On the ninth day of July, eighteen hundred and eighty six at a meeting of the Corporation of the Sisters of Charity

of the House of Providence, Vancouver W.T., it was agreed to purchase in the city of New Westminster, B.C. of Mrs. M. Howison Lots One (1) and Two (2) in Block 32 for the sum of four thousand dollars ($4,000).

> Sister Joseph of the S.H., Treasurer.
> Sister John of the Cross, Pres.[15]

The Sisters engaged architect and builder Thomas McKay as contractor. Born in Osgoode, Ontario, in 1842, McKay had left for California in 1867, then made his way to British Columbia ten years later. He and William Turnbull (1842–1912) had been responsible for the construction of the most important Catholic public buildings in New Westminster, including Saint Peter's Roman Catholic Church, Saint Ann's Academy and Saint Louis College.

An article published in the *Mainland Guardian* on July 21, 1886, shortly after the new hospital was announced, shows the broad support already received by Catholics at this time as it notes the work of Saint Joseph's Hospital in Victoria, the work of the Sisters of Saint Ann in helping children in New Westminster, and the record of the Sisters of Providence in providing hospitals in Portland, Spokane and Walla Walla. The article then encourages support for the hospital by saying that "the assistance of all good Christians on the mainland will be asked for this valuable undertaking," and it notes that the "patients of the hospital are not confined to any nationality or creed; they are offered to all alike, without distinction."[16]

When the Sisters of Providence arrived in August 1886 to begin the actual work on their new hospital, they were provided with accommodation by the Sisters of Saint Ann. Later they took up residence at "the old church, which had been transformed into living quarters."[17] This was almost certainly the old Saint Charles Native church.

Although much of the cost of building the hospital would eventually be secured through private loans from individuals, the Sisters counted primarily on donations. Among the first of these was $1,500 worth of land donated by the Oblates of Mary Immaculate and presented by Bishop d'Herbomez. But while the support of the Church and the people in the city of New Westminster was critical to the efforts to establish the hospital, it was the support of the working men on the railroads and in the mining and logging camps that would allow those efforts to culminate in success. As a result, on September 1, 1886, Sister Jean du Calvaire (Sister John of Calvary) and Sister Ethelbert, having fully canvassed the city for support, left New Westminster to solicit donations among the workers on the new Canadian Pacific Railway (CPR) spur line between Port Moody and New Westminster. Railroad construction was dangerous work, and almost one in ten men had died on the job in some areas as the line was pushed through the treacherous terrain of British Columbia. While the CPR had its own doctors and had even established one of its hospitals at Yale, BC, their hospitals were only large portable tents, so the Sisters took this opportunity to establish a working relationship with the railway's doctors, men such as Dr. John Matthew Lefevre, who had just begun work for the company. (Dr. Lefevre later practised in Vancouver at Saint Paul's Hospital, also established by the Sisters of Providence.) By the end of October on this first trip the Sisters had raised two thousand dollars.

At the same time as they were canvassing for donations, whenever time allowed, the Sisters operated a comprehensive medical outreach, serving as community nurses and going door to door to find those who were ill or needed treatment. Many of these people could not afford a doctor or a stay in a hospital. It was an incredible undertaking; not since the municipal council had canvassed the city to establish the need for a hospital in 1861 had anyone actually gone out to find who was in need and assist them.

In June 1886, as the plans were being drawn up for the Sisters of Providence's new hospital, the city of Vancouver, only incorporated a month earlier, burned to the ground after clearing fires got out of control. Many of the injured were transported to Royal Columbian Hospital in New Westminster or whatever place could hold them, illustrating the desperate

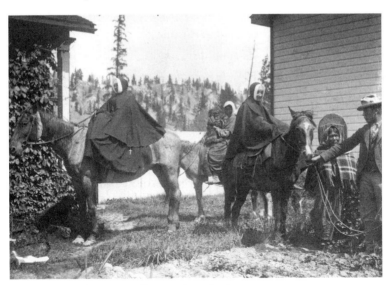

Sisters of Providence travelling on horseback. PHOTOGRAPH COURTESY OF NEW WESTMINSTER MUSEUM AND ARCHIVES MANUSCRIPT #302.

need for additional hospital and disaster capacity in the growing region.

During the fall of 1886 as the sisters continued their drive
to raise money for construction, the plans for the new hospital
were completed, the land was prepared and construction began.
Then on the night of January 15, 1887, the Arlington Hotel,
where architect and contractor Thomas McKay was staying,
caught fire. "The terrible calamity caused by this fire is unlike
anything ever known in this vicinity."[18] The fire started on the
ground floor and spread so quickly that the guests, some of
whom had lived in the hotel for months, lost everything they
owned. Were it not for the efforts of a Mr. Owens, who risked
his own life to alert and save many in the hotel, more would
have perished. In spite of his efforts, three men did die: 63-year-
old Mr. Campbell from Sherbrooke, Quebec, who had come
to New Westminster some months before with the intention of
establishing a woollen mill to produce cloth in the city; a Mr.
Brown of Huntingdon, Quebec; and Thomas McKay, who had
attempted to escape by jumping from a hotel window. But he
had tried to save himself too late. His clothing was already on
fire, and he died from his burns and injuries from his fall.

As a result, the very first use of the structure that was to
become Saint Mary's Hospital was as a morgue for the body of
McKay. A procession took McKay's body from there to Saint
Peter's church, which he had built himself, and laid him on
a platform in front of the altar as Oblate Father Paul Durieu
(who would become Bishop Durieu in 1890) held a solemn
mass. As McKay had been held in high esteem, and his prac-
ticality and building skills greatly valued in what was still a
pioneer city, the church was crowded. He was described by the

Mainland Guardian as "a thoughtful, prudent, peaceable citizen and a very clever man."[19] The large crowd made the march to the cemetery, led by Father Durieu, several other priests and all the Sisters in the city.

The loss of their architect and contractor was a huge blow to the Sisters of Providence. But they were also bereft for another reason: since McKay had used his hotel room as his office, the fire at the Arlington had also burned every important bit of paper related to the hospital's construction. The Sisters arranged for contractor J.B. Blanchet to come from Spokane to replace McKay on the job site, but Blanchet was not an architect, and work could not proceed until new plans were drawn up. The project was saved through the emergency intervention of the phenomenal Sister Joseph of the Sacred Heart, who came from Vancouver, Washington, to take charge and oversaw the completion of the hospital herself. Were it not for this timely involvement and the availability of such a talented individual, the death of Thomas McKay might well have been the end of Saint Mary's Hospital.

Construction costs amounted to $19,108.93 with another $1,165.53 spent on furnishings. The new hospital, which was also home to the Sisters of Providence, was a wood-frame, three-storey building eighty feet long and forty-five feet wide with the open wards common at the time, most likely with a curtain between each bed.[20] Although fireplaces were used inside the hospital, cooking and laundry facilities were housed in a separate building to minimize the risk of fire destroying the hospital. On April 27, 1887, as it was being constructed, the *Mainland Guardian* reported on some of the state-of-the-art elements that were being included in the building. A system of dumbwaiters allowed dinners to be taken hot up to the wards within half a minute of being prepared, a standard that would be difficult to achieve today. Water to the second floor was also worthy of note, and city residents who were lucky enough to be connected to the city's water supply found the "abundant supply of water" for the hospital's toilets to be something of a novelty. They were even more amazed to learn of the iron pipes that ran from the water tower in the yard along the building's

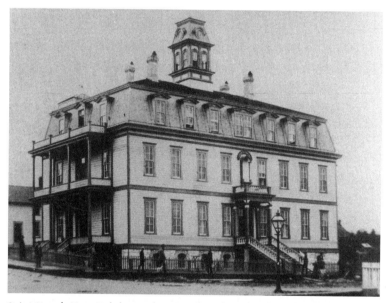

Saint Mary's Hospital, located at Agnes and Merrivale streets shortly after construction in 1887. In this photo of the original building, there is still construction debris near the fence to the right of the photo and a modern new gas lamp in front. There were no fire escapes at this time, but they would be added in later years, replacing the balconies that were built to allow patients easy access to fresh air and a spectacular view of the city and the river below. The small building to the rear likely held the laundry and cooking facilities, to minimize the risk of fire within the hospital. The hospital was formally opened on May 24, 1887. NEW WESTMINSTER MUSEUM AND ARCHIVES MANUSCRIPT #302.

ridgepole and gables in a kind of antique sprinkler system. In the event of fire, the opening of a faucet would cover the hospital instantly with water.

Saint Mary's Hospital opened its doors officially on May 24, 1887, the celebration having been delayed to coincide with Queen Victoria's birthday, and Father Durieu and other Oblate fathers officiated at the ceremonies.

3

The Great Builder

"As one of North America's early pioneer missionary nuns, Mother Joseph left a record of achievement that is an example to us all. Against great odds, along with other Sisters of Providence, she established hospitals and academic institutions, founded schools for Native children and homes for the elderly and infirm. Mother Joseph was the moving force behind the development of a large hospital system still in operation by the Sisters of Providence. She was indeed a woman worthy of her calling."

—PRIME MINISTER PIERRE ELLIOTT TRUDEAU,

OTTAWA, 1980

IN JANUARY 1887, the most important Sister of Charity of the House of Providence in the history of the Pacific Northwest, Mother Joseph of the Sacred Heart, arrived in New Westminster to complete the construction of Saint Mary's

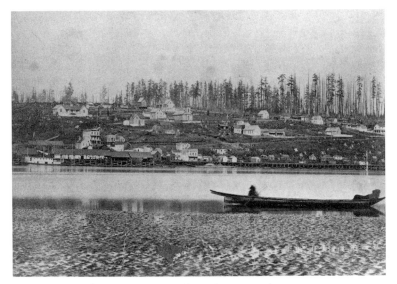

An early view of New Westminster from the Fraser River. PHOTOGRAPH
COURTESY OF NEW WESTMINSTER PUBLIC LIBRARY #279.

Hospital. It was not Mother Joseph's first hospital nor would it be her last work in New Westminster.

Although most widely known for her outstanding presence, both spiritual and temporal, Mother Joseph is also said to have had such an imposing height and solid build that she was easily recognizable even in her black nun's habit. Her perfectionism was legendary. Her buildings would not be shoddy and quick frontier constructions; with good humour but steady insistence she demanded quality and, as a result, her hospitals, schools and orphanages were built to last. She bounced on planks, hammered nails and climbed up into rafters. On one occasion when workmen improperly laid a chimney, she dismantled it and reassembled it correctly herself. At the age of sixty-four she lived in a shack at the construction site of one of her hospitals in order to keep a sharp eye on the work, not an unusual thing for her to do over her forty-six years of building social institutions. Yet Mother Joseph considered her determination to be a bit of a burden and would do penance for her self-perceived stubbornness. She was exactly the right person to take over the completion of Saint Mary's Hospital.

Mother Joseph had arrived in Washington Territory from Montreal back in 1856 with four other Sisters of Providence. The trip had taken five long stormy weeks because they had to travel around South America, due to an epidemic that prevented the scheduled rail trip across Panama. (The famous canal had yet to be built.) This was actually the second effort of the Sisters of Providence to establish badly needed services in the West. They had been forced to turn back in 1852, so this

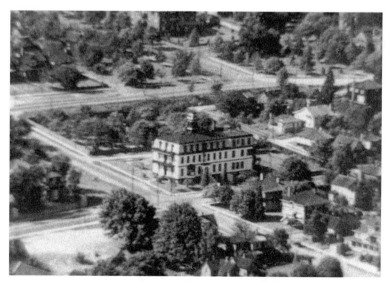

The hospital that Mother Joseph built. An early aerial photo of Saint Mary's Hospital. PHOTOGRAPH COURTESY OF SAINT MARY'S HEALTH FOUNDATION.

time they were determined not to fail. But, when they finally arrived in Fort Vancouver on December 8, they did not receive a warm welcome. Although in both 1852 and 1856 the Sisters had been invited to come west by Bishop Magloire Blanchet of Nesqually, Washington Territory, he had been away in Mexico when they arrived the first time and he was away in Europe when they arrived four years later. He had ordered the construction of a convent and schoolhouse for the Sisters, but his order had been countermanded by a vicar-general who wanted them to be based in Olympia. Infrequent mail exchanges, at only twice per year, are generally blamed for the lack of a resolution in this difference of opinion before the arrival of the Sisters. Without their host to greet them, the Sisters, after having endured such a long, hazardous journey and speaking only French in an English-speaking community, found scant welcome. They were gruffly assigned to an old and cluttered ten-foot by sixteen-foot attic, but it was here that they rose above difficulty and despair to establish their first headquarters, setting the tone for all the work of the Sisters of Providence in the West for the following years. They would remain self-sufficient, undertaking their own projects and staying firmly in control from start to finish.

Mother Joseph was almost a born carpenter. Christened Esther Pariseau at her birth on April 16, 1823, in Saint Elzear, near Montreal, she was the daughter of a carriage-maker who, recognizing her aptitude, had taught her carpentry from the time she was a child. In those days, however, a Catholic order was one of the few ways she could be allowed to use these skills professionally, so as a young woman she went to Montreal to join the Sisters of Charity of the House of Providence.

Thus, within days of finding herself and her companions in a cold attic in Fort Vancouver, this remarkable woman had transformed it into a combined dormitory and community room with a small temporary classroom. Then in February 1857, despite tensions over the Catholic presence in the area, the Sisters received their first property for a convent at Fort Vancouver—an old fur-storage building that was being used as a barn. Having fashioned her first headquarters out of an attic, Mother Joseph was undaunted by the task of creating a spiritual centre in a barn, although she did comment in a letter to the Superior General in Montreal that "beginnings are always trying, and here the devil is so enraged he frightens me."[21] She designed the chapel herself and with her own hands built the altar with a tabernacle made from an old candle box.

The first complex of the Sisters in Fort Vancouver developed much by accident. Although their intention in coming to the Pacific Northwest had not been to build hospitals but to build a school, needy children started to arrive before their school could be built. First, three-year-old Emily Lake, an orphan, was brought to the Sisters. Then a tiny baby boy was left on their doorstep. Soon Native children who were refugees and orphans from the Yakima Indian wars arrived at the Fort seeking care, and that task fell to the Sisters. Mother Joseph's construction skills easily dealt with the need. She built six small cabins and surrounded them with a picket fence. This small but growing complex became known as the "Providence suburb" of Fort Vancouver, its population of twenty-two souls consisting of five Sisters, two orphans, two boarding students, ten day students, and three elderly people who needed care.

The inspiration for the Sisters' first hospital came from the obvious need of an ordinary person, John Lloyd, a young man who was desperately ill with tuberculosis but had no permanent home. The Sisters nursed him and then others like him, but they had no place to house them, and taking in the needy to care for them was what the Sisters of Providence most actively sought to accomplish. According to histories of the Sisters' early days here, the idea of constructing a hospital was proposed by the local priest, and Mother Joseph, having already built a dormitory and classroom out of an attic and a convent out of a fur-storage barn, and now busily engaged in building a combined laundry and bakery, simply converted her new partially constructed building into a small hospital. When finished, it had two storeys and four beds, four tables and four chairs, but it was the forerunner to the order's Saint Joseph's Hospital, the first of the two dozen health centres she would build in the Pacific Northwest over the next forty-six years.

As an order, the Sisters of Providence were generally not wealthy in terms of cash, and only rarely could they independently finance their institutions, although each hospital, orphanage and school had to be self-sufficient. At one point, Mother Joseph wrote a letter to headquarters in Montreal, requesting the contribution of a spinning wheel so that the Sisters could save money by spinning their own wool. But while the Sisters managed to secure land and Mother Joseph found the ways and means to get her hospitals and orphanages built, maintaining and financing them after they were built was another matter entirely. And when local fundraising was not sufficient, it was Mother Joseph who came up with the idea of visiting local mining camps, catching the miners before they rushed to the saloons and brothels. She wrote about one of the earliest of these trips: "Finally, the trying ordeal of eighteen days in the saddle, extremely fatigued from the difficult days of travel, the long absence from home, camping under the heavens, on river banks and in sagebrush, we weary travellers reached the province of the Holy Angels, October 15, 1866."[22]

While fundraising was essential to the success of the Sisters' projects, Mother Joseph, not wanting the order to lose sight of their mission to the poor and to the community at large, set the tone for dealing with the wealthy early on. There was considerable pressure to get her to agree to build a hospital in Portland, Oregon, where Ben Holladay, a wealthy and politically powerful businessman, had offered a site with a good house, the use of his personal physician and some funds to pay for the initial part of the construction. Mother Joseph was skeptical. She knew Holladay was undertaking developments on the east side of Portland to support his real estate holdings, and she realized that his offer of a hospital site there neatly matched his ambitions to develop the area and increase his property values, but it would do nothing to serve any spiritual or health-care need of the existing population of Portland, which was mainly on the west side of the city. Added to this was the developer's reputation for questionable business practices and shady involvement in politics. Mother Joseph would have none of it. "She was unmoved by his charm or his claim to be Catholic."[23]

Always willing to bide her time to do things right as she saw them and determined to serve the needs of the community and not this real estate developer, Mother Joseph successfully found a site on the west side of the city where the people actually lived. The Society of Saint Vincent de Paul, a lay group, came forward with a $1,000 donation, no strings attached. Mother

Joseph drew up the plans for Saint Vincent Hospital herself, inspected the work regularly, and carved the wooden statue of the hospital's patron saint at its entrance herself. The doors were opened on July 18, 1875. From then on, the Sisters would place great importance on being independent from the wealthy land barons so that such considerations would not interfere with their spiritual mission and their commitment to health care for the local people. Positive relations with the community and with governments were also very important to the Sisters, but when there was a need to oppose the government, Mother Joseph was willing. When the town of Vancouver, Washington, decided to impose a water tax on her academy and sent a bill, she announced that she would dig her own well, and she did exactly that.

Some persons have been celebrated for having been the

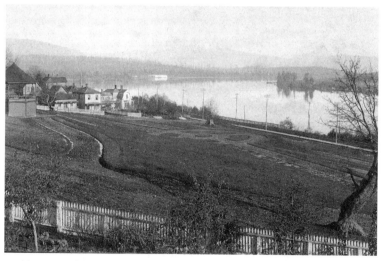

Looking onto the Fraser River from Albert Crescent. Saint Mary's was nearby and had a similar view. Circa 1890. PHOTOGRAPH BY S.J. THOMPSON, COURTESY OF NEW WESTMINSTER MUSEUM AND ARCHIVES IHP-0312.

founders of a single school or a single hospital, or simply for being the figurehead of a founding organization. Mother Joseph of the Sacred Heart of the Sisters of Providence did it all—she was architect, fundraiser, builder and artist. She was involved in every aspect of each construction, and she is officially credited with the design and construction of twenty-nine separate institutions. Saint Mary's Hospital is not counted in this list as she stepped in late to complete it. One of her last projects was also in New Westminster; thirteen years after the opening of Saint Mary's Hospital, she was responsible for the construction of Providence Orphanage, a beautiful four-storey brick building on a twelve-acre site on New Westminster's Twelfth Street. It opened in 1900 and, for the next fifty-nine years, provided care for British Columbia's orphans, only being phased out of operation when at last the provincial government assumed greater responsibility for the children. The building was demolished in 1960 and the land sold.

Although Mother Joseph's accomplishments included projects in Washington, Oregon, Idaho, Montana, and British Columbia, in 1901, in one of the final acts in her life, she encouraged the Sisters to go to California and establish a hospital in Oakland. She died in January 1902 of cancer. Those present at her death reported that her final words were "Sisters, whatever concerns the poor is always our affair."[24] Her close friend, Mother Mary Antoinette, wrote, "She had the characteristics of genius: incessant works, immense sacrifices, great undertakings; and she never counted the cost to self. She exercised an extraordinary influence on the Church in the West."[25]

As a builder of so many early social-service institutions, Mother Joseph may well be the most significant pioneer

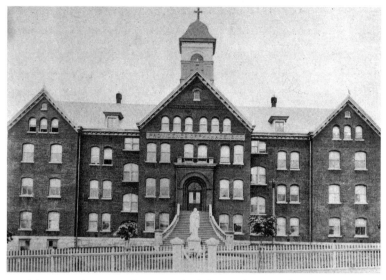

Providence Orphanage, circa 1932, built by Mother Joseph in 1900, as seen from the street. IMAGE B-09755 COURTESY OF ROYAL BC MUSEUM, BC ARCHIVES.

contributor to the Pacific Northwest, but while never a celebrity or public figure in life, after her death she was nearly forgotten in the United States and remains largely unknown in Canada. She was briefly remembered in 1953 when the American Institute of Architects declared her "The First Architect in the Northwest." Later, because of her early use of Douglas fir for wood carving, the West Coast Lumberman's Association declared her to be "the first white woman to work with wood in the Pacific Northwest," but her artistic output also included wax works and elaborate embroidery.

The life of Mother Joseph might still have been forgotten had it not been for a campaign to remember her started by historian Ann King after the Sisters of Providence announced plans to sell and demolish Providence Academy in Vancouver,

Washington. King tended Mother Joseph's grave and began organizing memorial efforts and programs such as nativity scenes at Christmas using a wax image of Jesus that had been hand-carved by Mother Joseph and adorned with snippets of hair from a young orphan who had once been cared for by the Sisters. The city supported King's campaign to avoid demolition and supported her efforts to find a buyer truly interested in the historic importance of the site. Finally it was purchased by Robert Hidden whose direct ancestor had made the bricks for the building. Meanwhile, King went ahead with the restoration of the chapel and the establishment of a memorial room to Mother Joseph.

The efforts of Ann King and her little group to have the life of Mother Joseph remembered and celebrated culminated on May 1, 1980, when, in the rotunda of the United States Capitol, House Speaker Thomas P. "Tip" O'Neil and the president pro tem of the United States Senate, Warren G. Magnuson, received into the National Statuary Hall the bronze statue of Mother Joseph presented by the State of Washington.[26] Fewer than a hundred Americans are commemorated in this manner, each state being permitted to select only two persons to be

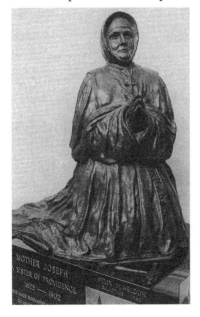

Mother Joseph Statue, US Capitol.
PHOTOGRAPH COURTESY OF THE US CAPITOL.

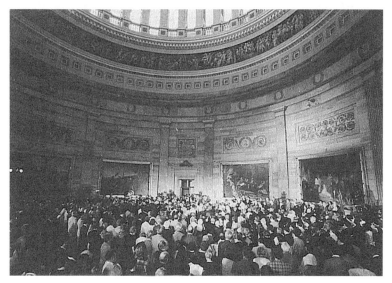

Dedication Ceremony for Mother Joseph Statue, US Capitol. PHOTOGRAPH
COURTESY OF THE US CAPITOL.

so honoured. She is the only Catholic Sister represented, the
only Canadian, and only the fifth woman. Her statue stands
in the rarest of company with those of just three former presi-
dents who have been chosen by their states—James Garfield of
Ohio, Andrew Jackson of Tennessee and George Washington
of Virginia.

Although Canadians remain largely oblivious to Mother
Joseph's historic importance, the Canadian anthem was played
at the ceremony, and Senator Ray Perrault, then leader of the
Canadian Senate, represented Canada along with the Canadian ambassador to the US. Prime Minister Pierre Trudeau sent
a letter, as did US President Jimmy Carter. A duplicate statue
can be seen in the state capitol at Olympia, Washington. The
sculptor was the renowned Felix de Weldon, who created the

famous monument to the raising of the US flag on Iwo Jima and several other significant monuments in Washington, DC.

Although French-speaking and born in Quebec, Mother Joseph of the Sacred Heart was honoured by Washington's Governor Dixy Lee Ray as "a great Washingtonian and a great American."[26] No such recognition of her important historic role has been made in British Columbia, even in New Westminster, which was the focus of her work in this province. Mother Joseph herself would likely not have sought any such recognition, but as Mike Haywood wrote in the *Columbian*, "Mother Joseph needs no monument but, as long as the niche is empty, it will be a monument to our forgetfulness."[27]

4

A Hospital for All

"As Servants of the Poor, have a true veneration for these suffering members of Jesus Christ . . . show that you love the poor by speaking of them always with esteem, finding your joy in helping them, using all the inventions of a tender charity to instruct them unto justice . . . in general prefer the care of the poor to the instruction of the rich . . . but above all prepare yourselves to be good nurses, good pharmacists, good visitors of the poor and the sick."

—BISHOP IGNACE BOURGET OF MONTREAL,
ADDRESSING THE SISTERS OF PROVIDENCE ON THEIR TWENTY-
FIFTH ANNIVERSARY, MARCH 25, 1868

THE NEWLY BUILT SAINT MARY'S HOSPITAL had forty-two beds and a staff of five Sisters, including Superior Sister John of Calvary, plus three employees. The hospital's first medical superintendent was one of the most exemplary physicians in early BC history. Doctor Charles Joseph Fagan (1857–1915)

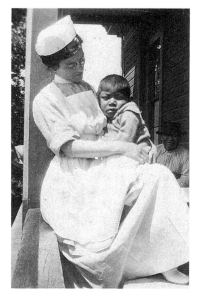

Nurse Ann Jackson and Native child, Saint Mary's Hospital, 1918.
PHOTOGRAPH COURTESY OF SAINT PAUL'S HOSPITAL ARCHIVES.

had graduated in medicine from Trinity College in Dublin, Ireland, and received his medical licence from Rotunda Hospital in Dublin in 1883. He practised in Staffordshire, England before emigrating to take the job with Saint Mary's. Later he formed a partnership with Dr. Richard E. Walker, which lasted until 1899 when he became secretary to the BC Board of Health. In this capacity he worked to introduce sanitary regulations in the fish-packing industry to control typhoid, and later was instrumental in the formation of the BC Anti-Tuberculosis Society and the establishment of the Tranquille Sanatorium near Kamloops. In 1908 he was elected president of the BC Medical Association.[28]

The first patient admitted to the new hospital on opening day, May 24, 1887, was a thirty-five-year-old Irish Catholic labourer named W. Cassidy of New Westminster. He was too poor to pay for his care, but far from being disappointed by this the Sisters were happy that they were succeeding in their mission to serve the poor. In fact, to begin the life of the hospital by caring for someone in such need was considered a very visible sign of God's work being done, and the Sisters were described as joyous at such a positive omen.

Expenses for the first full year of operation, July 1887–July 1888. By this time Saint Mary's had hired servants and was buying cows and chickens to supply the hospital with eggs and milk. The total bill for drugs for the hospital that year was $250.82. COURTESY OF NEW WESTMINSTER MUSEUM AND ARCHIVES MANUSCRIPT #302.

From this beginning, the Sisters proceeded to bring profound changes to the way hospitals were managed. Unlike the Royal Columbian, which did not accept children or persons with incurable conditions, Saint Mary's accepted both. And the Sisters did not discriminate by race. In some hospitals Chinese people would be segregated—that is, if the hospital was open to non-whites at all—and other hospitals had a policy of limiting the number of non-whites, so that if too many Japanese, for example, fell ill at once, those beyond the quota would not be admitted. As for the poor, some hospitals deliberately made their care as unpleasant as possible so they would not want to stay too long.

Several previous histories have stated that Saint Mary's had few patients in the early days and that most were old, one being over 100. In fact, the hospital records demonstrate that it was far more universal in its patient make-up than most hospitals of the time. Saint Mary's took in everyone—rough American prospectors, Japanese cannery workers, Chinese and Sikh labourers, Native people, Catholics and Protestants, the young, the old, the rich, the poor and the mentally ill. Even those who did not need medical care but were simply hungry were fed and sometimes clothed. It was the Sisters' mission to provide compassionate care for all, and that mission guided Saint Mary's policy from the first day of its existence and for all of its 117 years of service. However, it was from the beginning—as it would be for many decades—very much a hospital of the ordinary working man, partly because it was just uphill from the industrial area and wharves on the Fraser River, which made it very convenient to workers. In fact, almost three-quarters of those admitted in the early years were listed as labourers and, as a result, in 1887 the average patient age was just thirty-one, only seven patients were older than fifty and two were older than sixty-five. On the other hand, eight patients were under the age of nineteen, and five of those were aged five or under, including the youngest, one-year-old Albert E. Girard of Lulu Island, his four-year-old sister, Florence, and his five-year-old brother, Eugene.

Record keeping, of course, was not always precise in those days. A case in point is the Reverend Brother Allen who appears in Saint Mary's register twice in 1887; the first time he was listed as sixty years of age, the second time fifty-two. Perhaps there were two Reverend Brother Allens—which seems unlikely—or perhaps it is a testament to the healing power of Saint Mary's Hospital that he appeared to be eight years younger upon his second arrival. By the time he was admitted again in 1904 he was seventy. Added to the problem of keeping correct records was the fact that the Sisters' first language was French, they were keeping records in English, and patients were supplying information in a multitude of other tongues and from a wide array of cultures, many of which would have been completely unfamiliar to the recorder. Most of the Sisters would in time learn English, although for some it would remain a challenge.

Sometimes the problem with identification lay in the fact that different spellings were used for the same person's name, and sometimes information was obtained second-hand or even from someone who barely knew the patient. At other times people just did not know. A patient might have been baptized under one name and, being illiterate or perhaps never having seen a baptismal certificate, had used a different name or nickname all his life. And, in those days, it was not unusual for someone to be ignorant of his birth date as many births were never registered, and in large families it was not uncommon for the parents to forget to make a note of the date upon which there was yet another mouth to feed. Of course, some people just plain forgot how old they were or chose to fudge their ages a little for personal reasons.

But it is true that Saint Mary's did take in the old and infirm, something that many hospitals would not. While there is actually no record of any patient being over 100, Mrs. E. D'Aubignez of France was 83 years old—a remarkable age at that time—when she was admitted on September 3, 1887, for an unknown ailment. But there were many others, like the two unnamed senior patients admitted on July 19, 1888, who had no family or others to care for them in their senior years. For the young hospital, this kind of patient could pose a challenge as their stays could be long and they were generally unable to pay for their care and boarding. As an act of pure charity, therefore, the Sisters had to raise money and obtain donations in kind to sustain these elderly people to the end of their days. As a result, throughout its long years of service, Saint Mary's received loyalty from senior citizens grateful for the particularly kind and compassionate care for which the hospital became known from its earliest days.

A study of the patient register for Saint Mary's in the critical first year of operation is quite revealing. Between May 24, when the hospital opened, and December 26, when the last four patients of the year arrived, sixty-eight persons were admitted, fifty of them men and eighteen women. (This total does not count those patients seen in their homes and those who were treated but did not stay overnight in hospital.) The majority of these patients were not Catholic; in fact, just over half (thirty-five) were Protestant, demonstrating how Saint Mary's crossed the religious divide. And the Protestants admitted were not just working men. Over the years many of them were, like John Galbraith who was treated for consumption, members of the city's powerful business establishment or, like Mayor Thomas Ovens who had surgery there, leaders in the political community. And they often found themselves in bed next to someone of an entirely different faith. On July 21, 1891, the local Catholic priest Father Hackett was admitted suffering from "general debility" and, while the good priest was in hospital, J.M. Donaldson was admitted for rheumatism and stayed roughly three weeks. Donaldson was a minister of the Church of England. He could have chosen to go to the Royal Columbian, yet there he was with Father Hackett at Saint Mary's. And among the other patients there at that time was a certain Mr. Brung, a non-Catholic Japanese—most likely a Buddhist—who had been struck by lightning. These three men convalesced in the hospital together with other patients, most of them non-Catholics. This is the way it was at Saint Mary's Hospital. There may have been religious tensions and prejudice elsewhere, but the mission of Saint Mary's to provide compassionate health care meant that there was no discrimination when it came to caring for those in need.

Exactly half of the sixty-eight patients in the first year's patient register were from New Westminster, and some carried pioneer family names important to the city's history, such as McBride, Walford and Binnie. Others had surnames still well known in the Royal City today, such as McQuarrie, Crean and Winne. Nine of the first-year patients came from Lulu Island,

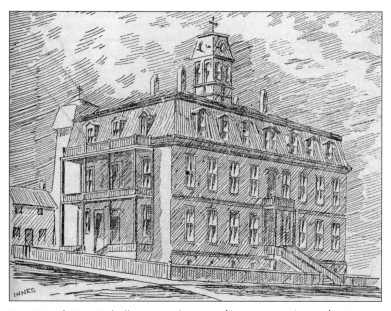

Saint Mary's Hospital. Illustration by Innes (first name unknown), 1892 City Directory. *HENDERSON'S BRITISH COLUMBIA GAZETEER*, 1892, COURTESY OF NEW WESTMINSTER PUBLIC LIBRARY.

and among that nine were two whole families, the Lindsays and the Girards. Patients also came from Lytton, Vancouver, Port Moody, Hurling Bay, Lillooet, Hope and Mud Bay, and one each from Oregon City and "Sanfrisco."

The ethnic diversity in that first year of operation is also striking: twenty-two patients were Irish, while only five were English. Eight were Scottish, two were German and one was French. The strong continuing American presence in the area, long after the Cariboo Gold Rush had peaked, is shown by the fact that sixteen Americans were admitted as patients, second in number only to the Irish, and it has been suggested that most of those Irish had actually arrived via the United States. Only six patients were described as Canadians, but, at that time, just twenty years after Confederation, most people in this country were still classified according to their national origin. At least three of those six Canadians were francophone. Saint Mary's also played an important role from the very beginning for the Native people of New Westminster as well as serving as the hospital for Saint Mary's Mission, upriver from New Westminster. Seven patients in the first year were described as "Indian" or "half breed," eighteen-year-old August Billy of New Westminster being typical of them.

Among all the groups represented in Saint Mary's patient register during the early years it is probably safe to say that only the French were attracted there by the fact that the Sisters of Providence were from Quebec (they referred to themselves as "Canadienne"). Of the 141 listed in Saint Mary's register as French during the first twenty years of the hospital's existence, seventy were specifically listed as having come from France, three from Acadia, two from Corsica, one from Quebec; the

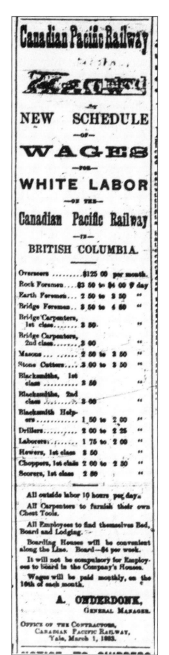

CPR advertisement for white labour.
MAINLAND GUARDIAN, FEBRUARY 13, 1884.

other sixty-five were simply listed as French.

French Canadians had arrived in British Columbia early, as many had worked for the North West and Hudson's Bay companies, at least 800 having been employed in the fur trade by 1850, and many of them helped to establish Fort Langley. Before the arrival of the Royal Engineers, British Columbia had been protected by the Voltigeurs, a military corps based in Victoria and made up mainly of francophones. In the west the Roman Catholic clergy were almost entirely French, with most of the male clergy actually coming directly from France. Locally the priesthood was dominated by the Oblates of Mary Immaculate, an order of priests who had arrived in Canada in 1841. The Cariboo Gold Rush had attracted more Frenchmen, and in the 1880s there was some effort to recruit French Canadians to build the railways before the railroad companies began emphasizing the recruitment of less expensive Chinese labourers. Then in 1909 the Fraser Mills Lumber Company brought forty families from Quebec and settled them at Westminster Junction, later known as Maillardville, in Coquitlam. These new residents could speak English at various levels of proficiency, though some had no English at all, so having a nearby hospital where the staff nurses could speak French was very welcome. As a result, in later years whenever public opinion was tested, Coquitlam residents would be polled as being even more supportive of Saint Mary's Hospital than were New Westminster residents. Maillardville continued to be predominantly French until the 1950s, and "l'hôpital Sainte-Marie" was effectively their community hospital.

However, if there is one group to which Saint Mary's owed much of its initial success and acceptance, it was to the Americans living in British Columbia. When the Sisters of Providence established Saint Mary's Hospital in 1887, their French background posed a significant challenge among the established English-speaking population. It was just a year after the Riel Rebellion, and many of the British colonials had developed virulently anti-French attitudes, so if the hospital had been forced to rely on their support it might not have succeeded. The Sisters had, therefore, turned to the miners and labourers in the local camps who were far more likely to be American than British.

There were good reasons why the Americans were partial to the new hospital, but they were an exact reversal of those that had influenced the American attitude when the Sisters of Providence had come west to Oregon Territory in the early years of settlement. At that time much of the population had resented them. They were considered foreigners, loyal to a distant and foreign Pope. Even those settlers who were not outright anti-Catholic still often resented the Church's support of the Native people in the area, whom they regarded, from their point of view at the time, as murderous savages. But the Oblate missionaries lost their welcome among the tribes when they were unable to stop US troops systematically massacring the Native people. At the same time, anti-Catholic American vigilantes were attacking the priests and their missions. Thus, when the Oblates moved north to British Columbia in 1858, it was effectively an evacuation.

But American attitudes toward Catholic missionaries began to change during the Civil War that raged in the United States from 1861 to 1865, just a little more than twenty years before Saint Mary's was built, because Catholic Sisters played a critical role in caring for the wounded on both sides of the dispute. The Sisters saw the terrible conditions that existed for the wounded, especially in the army field hospitals, "although these were actually fairly free from the infectious diseases that turned base hospitals into charnel houses. Amputation was, of course, the most frequent operation and was carried out on a wholesale scale, usually in the open and in sight of passersby and waiting patients. Patients arrived with maggots half-an-inch long in their wounds. Surgeons cut and sawed until their hands trembled with fatigue; men died as they waited their turn; doctors held their knives between their teeth in between operations and probed wounds with dirty fingers; flies swarmed everywhere; and after a big battle blood flowed so freely that the scene resembled a slaughter house rather than a hospital."[29] As most deaths in the Civil War were actually from diseases and infections rather than combat, in their own hospitals the nuns placed a high priority on detecting and treating infectious diseases. They also emphasized the importance of good food and good facilities to prepare and distribute meals to their patients, so that their hospitals were seen as far safer places than those maintained by the army.

Almost 600 Sisters from at least twelve different orders served as nurses in that war, and the Nuns of the Battlefield Monument that stands today in Washington, DC, is a tribute to their service. But while this involvement of the nursing Sisters helped to change the attitudes of Americans toward their own minority Catholic population, it also indirectly benefited the people of British Columbia when Saint Mary's Hospital opened its doors twenty years later under the care of Catholic Sisters. When the design for Saint Mary's was drawn up, it was based on the ward style popular during the Civil War, a style that accommodated large numbers of patients in times of emergency, and it was this feature that later allowed the hospital to provide effective relief in times of local disasters and epidemics. As well, the orchards, farm animals and gardens that the Sisters incorporated into the grounds of Saint Mary's were as much a response to their recent Civil War lessons about maintaining a constantly available and healthy food supply as they were to their need to save money.

While the American population in British Columbia had been insignificant before the gold rush began in 1858, in that single year some 30,000 gold seekers, most of them Americans, made their way up the Fraser River, at times resembling a great invasion fleet as they sailed past the site where New Westminster would be incorporated two years later. Their arrival caused something close to panic among the small colonial population, but as the years went by and the gold rush peaked and mining and miners became part of just another industry, the Americans who stayed on became an accepted part of the landscape. For many years, in fact, the biggest holidays on the mainland were the Queen's birthday and the Fourth of July.

What was different in the attitude of the Americans in New Westminster to the arrival of the Sisters of Providence and the attitude of the people in Oregon to the Sisters' arrival was partly that the Americans coming to BC were gold seekers rather than settlers. The prospectors weren't interested in driving out the Native people in order to farm their land, so the Sisters' services to the Native people were not seen as contrary to their interests. In addition, by the time the Sisters of Providence arrived in New Westminster in 1886, the Oblates had established their legitimacy with local authorities, in part through their success in converting Native people to Christianity. (This success didn't always win support among Europeans, particularly when it interfered with liquor sales, and at least one Oblate spreading the gospel of the sober life was attacked by a mob of liquor merchants.) But the most significant factor in the success of the Sisters of Providence among the Americans was their outreach work. By going door to door and visiting the mining, logging and work camps where many of them were employed, the Sisters were highly visible and they demonstrated that their work was not some sort of abstract idea or limited to the hospital in New Westminster. They quickly established support and legitimacy.

As a result, there were times in the early years of Saint Mary's when a majority of patients at the hospital were actually from the United States. They included people like Mr. Sparks, a thirty-two-year-old New Westminster labourer who suffered from delirium tremens in 1891, and Olive Jordan, a twenty-two-year-old prostitute suffering from syphilis in 1903. There is also the interesting case of a fifty-four-year-old labourer named Joseph Stevens or Stephens who was admitted on October 3, 1890, with a sprained ankle and remained in hospital until October 20. He returned on March 19, 1891, with a "cold" (probably bronchitis) that was bad enough for him to be hospitalized for four days, and he was back again on May 5, 1891, for eleven days with a sore ankle. The interesting thing about this man was that, although the Sisters normally recorded only the patient's country of origin, they listed him as "negro." However, this was an anomaly and it is likely that a number of the other patients who were listed as American were also black.

Chinese people had been part of the life of British Columbia from as early as 1788 when Captain John Meares brought Chinese artisans by ship to Nootka to help him build a new vessel. While there is a common perception that the first Chinese arrived to build the railway, in fact, the first wave of Chinese immigration was in 1858 when they came north from the California Gold Rush to join the Fraser River Gold Rush. But not all of them went on to the goldfields. The November 24, 1860, issue of the *New Westminster Times* noted that large numbers of Chinese were camped on Victoria Gardens, later to be the site of Holy Trinity Cathedral. A concentration of Chinese businesses was soon established along Front Street, and a Chinatown would also form in the west end of the city, an area sometimes known as "The Swamp" that was roughly between

Eighth and Tenth streets and between Royal Avenue and the waterfront. The Chinese population was mostly made up of male labourers who planned to make their fortunes and return to China, though over time increasing numbers settled permanently in the new land.

The construction of the CPR in the 1880s resulted in larger than usual numbers of Chinese labourers being brought into the province and, in 1882, just five years before Saint Mary's opened its doors, more than eight thousand of them arrived in BC, mostly from Hong Kong and San Francisco. According to a Royal Commission on Chinese Immigration in 1884, there were 1,680 Chinese in New Westminster. Most—86 percent— were labourers, half working on the railways or in the mines and half employed as cooks, servants, fish hands or store clerks. When the provincial government, alarmed at their growing numbers, subsequently tried to ban the immigration of Chinese, the federal government disallowed the law. In 1885, however, the federal government was persuaded to impose a "head tax" of $50 on Chinese immigrants and this slowed immigration in the next few years. In addition, both civic and provincial governments took measures to limit the use of Chinese labour, including barring employers of Chinese

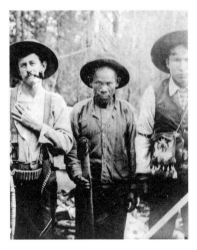

Chinese gold miner Ah Bau, circa 1858. IMAGE A-04279 COURTESY OF ROYAL BC MUSEUM, BC ARCHIVES.

from obtaining city contracts or from accessing city equipment.

After the Knights of Labour started an anti-Asian riot in Vancouver on February 23, 1887, most of that city's Chinese relocated to New Westminster, and for many years New Westminster had the largest Chinese population on the British Columbia mainland. By this time health conditions were already very poor in the overcrowded Chinese district, and although local residents did seek improvements from the city, all too often city officials ignored them or blamed the Chinese themselves, hoping that the rundown state of the area would drive them away. In time it became a breeding ground for typhoid, as well as many other diseases. In 1886 the Knights of Labour approached city council to express their concern after several cases of leprosy were reported in Chinatown. And on November 16, 1901, Saint Mary's dealt with a case of bubonic plague when thirty-seven-year-old Chinese labourer Woo Wing died there of the disease. He had recently arrived from San Francisco where an epidemic of the plague had just broken out.

The Chinese were the least likely of New Westminster's residents to use western medical services as they preferred their own traditional remedies and practices. Most of them avoided surgery at all costs, even when death threatened, in the belief that a body that was not whole in life would not be whole in the afterlife. Better to suffer for a little while now than for all of eternity. When Chinese people did seek medical help, they came to Saint Mary's because it was the closest general hospital to the city's Chinatown. The first Chinese patient, simply recorded as a "Chinaman" from China, was admitted to Saint Mary's Hospital on March 11, 1888; he was a labourer and

MUNICIPAL COUNCIL.

The Council met on Monday night: Present—His Worship the Mayor.—Couns. Douglas, Benson, Elliott, Shiles, Calbick, and Lord.

The minutes of the last meeting were read and approved.

The master workman of the Knights of Labour calls the attention of the Council to the necessity of removing the Chinese lepers.

To the Mayor and Council.

We, the local assembly of the Knights of Labor respectfully draw your attention to the fact that there are several cases of leprosy amongst the Chinese of this city, and we believe it is your duty to protect the citizens from this disease. The persons diseased not only infest the savoury abodes of China town, but enter the houses of citizens and exhibit their sores for the purpose of obtaining alms.

ALEXANDER HAMILTON,
Master Workman,
W. W. FORESTER Secty.

Coun. Lord—I propose that the Knights of Labor be requested to employ a doctor who will report to us.

Coun. Benson—I move that the Knights be requested to mind their own business.

Coun. Shiles seconded the motion of Coun. Lord and it was carried.

The Knights of Labour approached New Westminster City Council about cases of leprosy in the Chinese community. *MAINLAND GUARDIAN*, SEPTEMBER 8, 1886.

he died that same day. When city council demanded that all city establishments refuse to hire or even serve the Chinese community, Saint Mary's, unlike other hospitals, simply carried on as usual and kept its doors open to them. It was, however, a decision destined to cause a rift between the Sisters and women's groups in the city who supported discrimination against the Chinese population.

However, the fact that any of New Westminster's Chinatown residents came to be served by Saint Mary's Hospital at all was due in large part to one man, Won Alexander Cumyow.

Some typhoid cases as recorded in the hospital's register. Patient Register, 1887—1907. COURTESY OF NEW WESTMINSTER MUSEUM AND ARCHIVES MANUSCRIPT #302.

Born March 27, 1861, at Fort Douglas, he is generally regarded as the first person of Chinese descent born in Canada. His
father had a business supplying miners entering the goldfields,
and Won Cumyow learned to speak Chinook from the Native
people who visited his father's store. When the family moved
to New Westminster after the gold rush ended, Won Cumyow
attended school there along with the notoriously anti-Asian
politician Richard McBride, premier of British Columbia from
1903 to 1915. Won Cumyow was the first Chinese Canadian
to study law at UBC and even to article, but he could not enter
the bar as he was not on the voters list, the Chinese in Canada
having been disenfranchised in 1875.

Since he was skilled in several Chinese dialects and English as well as Chinook, and because he had studied law, in

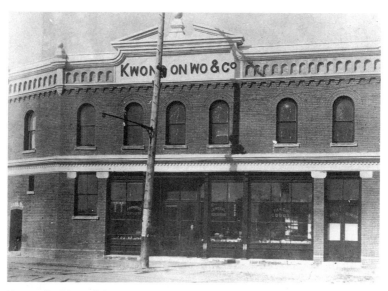

Kwong On Wo and Company, Front Street, New Westminster. The sign on
the left behind the pole advertises "Prepared Opium." PHOTOGRAPH COURTESY
NEW WESTMINSTER PUBLIC LIBRARY.

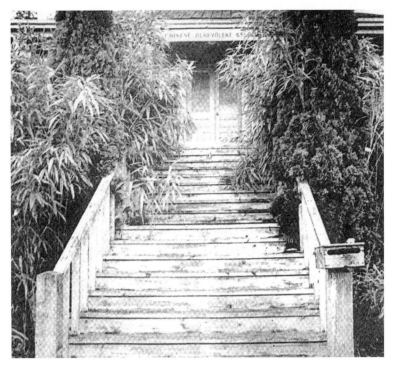

The former Chinese Hospital in 1979, as it was when donated to the City of New Westminster, shortly before being demolished. The sign, in English, of the Chinese Benevolent Association, can be easily read. Among the plants is bamboo from the original Chinese garden. *THE COLUMBIAN*, JULY 24, 1979, COURTESY OF NEW WESTMINSTER PUBLIC LIBRARY.

1888 Won Cumyow was hired as the first court interpreter in New Westminster's history; he served in the same capacity in Vancouver from 1904 to 1936. As a result of his official position between cultures and his involvement in the Chinese Benevolent Society and the Empire Reform Association, he became a significant leader in the Chinese communities of both cities. And being a strong supporter of western health care, he was able to convince other Chinese to accept modern medicine and make use of local hospitals. He supported even those hospitals that discriminated against Chinese patients, and he raised thousands of dollars for the Vancouver General, despite that hospital's policy of restricting Chinese patients to the basement, a policy that remained in effect until 1920. He was a patient in Saint Mary's himself in October 1904 and was largely responsible for the fact that the numbers of Chinese coming to Saint Mary's for treatment increased steadily over the years. (The many long years of service that the Sisters of Providence provided to the Chinese community was rewarded on August 3, 1962, when Mr. Nip Fong donated 83 acres of timberland on Vancouver Island to the hospital.)

Although many Chinese continued to come to Saint Mary's, in 1905 the Chinese Benevolent Society undertook the construction of a hospital at 835 Agnes Street, surrounding it with a garden that included a grove of wild bamboo. Like many of the early hospitals, this building served a variety of purposes over the years while continuing to function as a small hospital.

Yearly No. 171	**S. BOWELL & SON** NEW WESTMINSTER, B.C. Book____ Page____ Month December Case No. 2

NAME OF DECEASED — W O N G   L O Y   (Wong Yeu Yow)
ADDRESS — New Westminster, B.C.
DIED AT — Chinese Hospital, Agnes St., New West'r. DATE OF DEATH December 2, 1934.
SEX Male   RACIAL ORIGIN Chinese   MARRIAGE STATE Married.   10:00 A.M.
BIRTHPLACE — China.
DATE OF BIRTH — April 14, 1876.   AGE 58-7-18.
OCCUPATION — Farmer.
PLACE OF BURIAL — Mountain View Cemetery.   DATE OF FUNERAL December 4, 1934.
MINISTER — - - -   LOCATION OF GRAVE
PHYSICIAN — Dr. O. Van Etter.
CAUSE OF DEATH — Myocarditis.

ORDERED BY — Wong Ling,   CHARGE TO Wong Ling,
ADDRESS — 48 McInnes St., City.   48 McInnes St., City.

The funeral card of Wong Loy, or Wong Yeu Yow, who died at the Chinese Hospital in 1934 and was buried at Mountain View Cemetery. BOWELL FUNERAL HOME RECORDS, COURTESY OF NEW WESTMINSTER PUBLIC LIBRARY.

At various times, it also housed the Chinese School and the Benevolent Association, and in its later years, when most of the patients were elderly men, it came to be known as the Chinese Old Men's Home. In the 1970s the building—now one of the oldest in the downtown area—was given to the city as a gift. But nine years later—at a time when there was less knowledge and awareness of history, particularly ethnic history—the city demolished it.

The history of the Japanese community in British Columbia began in New Westminster in 1877 when Manzo Nagano jumped ship and became the first Issei. Over the next few decades the Japanese community grew and prospered, and although many settled throughout the Fraser Valley, one of the main enclaves was in Steveston where the Japanese fishermen built a small hospital primarily to house those suffering

Yearly No. 169	S. BOWELL & SON NEW WESTMINSTER, B.C.	Book	Page
		Month November	Case No. 13

NAME OF DECEASED	Y U E S A E L I N G .		
ADDRESS	Shanghai, China. (S.S.City of Victoria)		
DIED AT	St. Mary's Hospital, New Westminster, B. C.	DATE OF DEATH November 26/34,	12;35
SEX Male	RACIAL ORIGIN Chinese	MARRIAGE STATE Married	a.m.
BIRTHPLACE	China		
DATE OF BIRTH	1879	AGE 55 years	
OCCUPATION	Chief Steward.		
PLACE OF BURIAL	shipped to Shanghai, China.	DATE OF shipment January 12, 1935	
MINISTER	---	LOCATION OF GRAVE	
PHYSICIAN	Dr. W. A. Clarke.		
CAUSE OF DEATH	Chronic Myocarditis. (Contributory-- Syphilis.)		
ORDERED BY	Ocean Shipping Co.,	CHARGE TO	
ADDRESS			
Shipped on board S. S. Empress of Canada.			
Shipped to C. W. Gordon, 12 The Bund, Shanghai, China.			

This funeral home record shows that the body of Yue Sae Ling, who died at Saint Mary's Hospital on November 26, 1934, was shipped back to China because most Chinese preferred to be buried close to their ancestors. Chinese charities often raised funds for this, and some exhumation took place when the money was available to repatriate the bodies.
BOWELL FUNERAL HOME RECORDS, COURTESY OF NEW WESTMINSTER PUBLIC LIBRARY.

from infectious diseases. In New Westminster, Japanese people settled in Queensborough and in the old Chinatown. In fact, Chinatown was about half Japanese by the time the Japanese were interned in 1942.

However, even after the small Japanese hospital opened, Saint Mary's continued to serve as the primary hospital to the Japanese community because of its excellent track record in dealing with typhoid and in welcoming Japanese patients. The first person from Japan listed in Saint Mary's patient register was twenty-nine-year-old Tiny Goodsy, a fisherman, who was admitted suffering from fever in September 1889 and stayed for thirteen days. But he would not be the last Japanese fisherman to enter Saint Mary's Hospital with a fever. As with most of the hospital's patients, those working for the canneries had the usual run of injuries, but for the fishermen the real threat was typhoid. Between 1887 and 1907 typhoid and other fevers made up roughly 60 percent of all hospital admissions of Japanese patients. Of the typhoid victims, about two-thirds were fishermen working on the river and the rest were labourers at the canneries.

For the next two decades, typhoid outbreaks on the river were an annual summer event, and as Saint Mary's became the preferred hospital of the Japanese communities, the Sisters bore the brunt of their care through each epidemic. However, Japanese patient numbers also increased because the wealthy cannery owners, men such as Alexander Ewen and Marshall English (one of the hospital's most prominent American supporters), arranged contracts with the hospital to provide medical care as part of an overall strategy to secure a stable and reliable workforce. Thus, when the thirty-two-year-old Japanese "Brung" survived a lightning strike at English's Cannery, his care was all covered under the cannery's medical plan with Saint Mary's.

Although the first patient to enter Saint Mary's on its very first day of operation was the Irishman, Mr. Cassidy, he had been quickly followed by Mrs. A.B. Clark, aged twenty-nine, and Miss H. Clark, aged five, both of them Native people from Lytton. Mrs. Clark died on June 6, 1887, in all probability leaving the child as the first orphan to be cared for by the Sisters. In the years to come, Saint Mary's would become the primary hospital for Saint Mary's Mission, the Good Shepherd Orphanage and Providence Orphanage, all of which had large numbers of young Natives in their care.

However, even before Saint Mary's was built, the Catholic Church had a long and positive relationship with the First Nations communities in British Columbia, going back to the 1860s when Father Fouquet vaccinated three thousand Native people against smallpox, thereby encouraging many of them to become converts. The importance of aboriginal converts was also shown in 1864 when Bishop d'Herbomez, the first Catholic bishop of British Columbia, was installed, and the ceremony took place at New Westminster's Saint Charles Church. It had been built especially for services in the Chinook language after the local Native leaders forbade the Catholic priests to preach to their people unless they spoke Chinook, and the priests had set about learning the language. It was only after Saint Charles Church fell into disuse, having been superseded by Saint Mary's Mission (farther up the Fraser River) as the centre of First Nations religious life, that the use of Chinook became less of an issue. However, the rule was still a reality when Saint Mary's Hospital was built in 1887, and several of the Sisters made the effort—with various levels of proficiency—to communicate in that language. It may have also had an effect on the new hospital's construction: according to an early article in the *Mainland Guardian*, when Saint Mary's was built, a small "Indian hospital," financed by funds raised by the Native community, was also constructed on the site. As neither the Oblates nor the Sisters of Providence supported segregation, it seems possible that this building was constructed in order to keep Native patients separate where they could communicate with the nursing staff in Chinook. There is, however, no other information available about this Native hospital.

When the Sisters of Providence arrived, the aboriginal population had been decimated by disease. A smallpox epidemic in 1836–38 had taken the lives of approximately a third of their population on the coast; an epidemic in 1860–62, twenty-five years before Saint Mary's opened, had taken another nineteen thousand lives. The survivors were far worse off than second-class citizens. They had no citizenship to speak of, and governments had reneged on most of the agreements to provide them with land reserves and support. The attitude displayed by Dr. William Fraser Tolmie in his journal for 1835 was enlightened compared with what would come in later years:

Thursday January 22: Wacash who has been affected with a vomiting of blood for some days past came last night and applied for medicine, but fearing that should he die and his friends might demand payment as is the custom in the interior of the Columbia, I would give him nothing. Boston today pleaded hard in his behalf, but without effect. In the afternoon Wacash departed, in all likelihood offended. It is a pity that the prejudices of the natives oblige one to withhold assistance, where it would probably be of some service.[30]

Although the medicine of the aboriginal people contained many elements of song, spirit beliefs, and other non-scientific practices, many of the remedies they used were effective. However, after Christian denominations branded Native cultural practices as superstitious and pagan, the government outlawed and suppressed them. After that, while Native medicine did survive in some quarters, it could not be practised openly, and as a result much knowledge was lost. Had Europeans been more open, they might have learned that Native people were already successfully practising surgery (including trephining) and making use of fish oil for burns. Thus, although the Native people came to accept western medicine, they often still preferred the best of both worlds.

Many of the aboriginal patients in the registers of Saint Mary's Hospital were listed as "half-breed," reflecting government policy that only "full blood" Native people were qualified to have their hospitalization paid for by the federal government. Since almost half of all Saint Mary's Native patients between 1887 and 1907 were listed as "half-breed," this placed a large burden on the Sisters to find the money to cover their hospitalization and medical care. At the same time there is no doubt that the federal government had confidence in the care given to Native people at Saint Mary's as the local Indian agent, A. Baker, was hospitalized there with a broken leg for five weeks in 1903.

Over the years, hundreds of aboriginals were served by Saint Mary's, partly because much of the Native population in the earliest days was migratory, arriving in New Westminster to trade during warmer weather. Later Native people would supply much of the labour force on the river, and Saint Mary's longtime role as the hospital for the river workers and the hospital of local aboriginals would coincide.

From the beginning, the hospital's wards were a cacophony of accents and languages, and every day the Sisters took care of people from all over the world. German, Irish, Scottish and English patients were common, but there were also Dutch, Italian, Swiss, "Pollish," Portuguese, Russian and Australian, and the hospital seemed to be very popular with the small Greek community. There were even a couple of Corsicans, and a "Meulatto." The records list a few Spanish-speaking patients from Central America and Chile and several from Spain itself. With so many groups, people and languages in the hospital

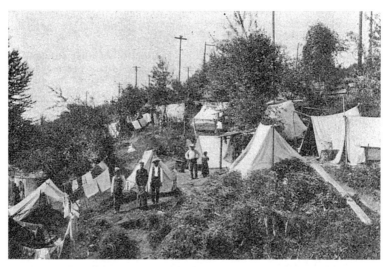

This was likely a fishing camp. Native patients at Saint Mary's Hospital tended to increase in the summer months when many arrived in the area for the fishing season. *THE COAST MAGAZINE,* OCTOBER 1905.

wards, Saint Mary's was positively Bohemian. In fact, in 1889 Frank Koal, a local farmer, was admitted suffering from fever and his nationality was duly recorded—Bohemian! As a result of this mixture of people, medical care was often delivered through a translator—if one could be found.

On February 19, 1900, a typical day at Saint Mary's, a fisherman from Finland named A. Harrickson, who had been admitted with a sore leg, was about to be released. He left behind in the ward Wo Haa and Sing Woo, two Chinese labourers who had received cuts to the head. William Mathens, an Australian labourer living in Sapperton, was being treated for blood poisoning. An unnamed Japanese labourer from Sapperton and Alexander Reid, a Scottish labourer living in New Westminster, were suffering from "cold." Alex Innes, a Scot who lived in the Power House, had typhoid fever. Because of his contagious disease, Innes might have been kept in a separate room, but the others would have shared a common ward, their beds next to each other, without segregation or concern about race or ethnicity.

On May 16, 1905, L. Ketas, a three-year-old New Westminster boy, arrived as a patient, his profession dutifully entered into the patient register as "baby." What ailed him is not known but he stayed for three days so perhaps he was one of the many victims of the life-threatening bouts of flu common at the time. There is not much else of note about young little L. Ketas, except for one thing: under the heading "nationality" is the word "Jewish." Then there was the "Hindoo" man who suffered from the flu for four days in February 1907. Communicating with him was likely a problem as his name and country were not recorded, but he was a resident of New Westminster and received care without question at Saint Mary's.

In April 1888 Saint Mary's staff began recording the ailments of patients. There were numerous examples of infectious diseases, including typhoid, as well as serious accidents, primarily involving labourers. These included an amputation for a twenty-seven-year-old New Westminster man named A.E. Fraser, who then spent three months in hospital, and twenty-one-year-old Ed Donald from Saint Mary's Mission, who had been shot. He died the day he was admitted, October 7, 1888. Patients were also admitted suffering from such things as "hurt," fatigue, "drink," old age, paralysis, broken bones, weakness, general debility, sore joints and other matters simply recorded as "private."

The tendency of the Sisters of Providence to build their hospitals in the centres of population also meant that they were the closest to the poor who gathered in urban areas. Thus, while primarily built to minister to the sick, Saint Mary's also came to the aid of those in need as the result of other circumstances, including abandonment, loss of family and hunger. One twenty-two-year-old woman was brought to the hospital in June 1887 after her husband was sentenced to life in prison. She and her youngest child were allowed to stay at the hospital, while her three other daughters stayed with the Sisters of Saint Ann.

Even with the Provincial Hospital for the Insane located in the community—or perhaps because of it—Saint Mary's admitted many mentally ill persons on compassionate grounds. There were patients such as Mrs. Mulhall of Vancouver, aged thirty-six, who was admitted for three months in 1889 for "insanity." The hospital even played an early role in treating alcoholism, as in the case of a Mr. McNaulty, aged seventy-five, of New Westminster who received care for one month in 1888 when he was suffering from the ailment of "drink." Saint Mary's also admitted patients diagnosed with melancholy, depression and "general debility." The kind care provided to such patients contrasted sharply with the scandals at the asylum, and Saint Mary's Hospital continued to receive patients with mental illness and addictions for many decades.

But not only did the poor and the sick come to the hospital, the hospital also came to them. The Sisters made visits to homes in "The Swamp" in the city's west end and in the forested areas around the city, as well as throughout the Fraser Valley and in the work camps of the province, thus becoming, when this outreach is considered, the most important health institution in the province. In fact, in its first full year of operation, it is estimated that the Sisters operating out of Saint Mary's Hospital rendered compassionate assistance on more than three thousand occasions. Often they discovered desper-

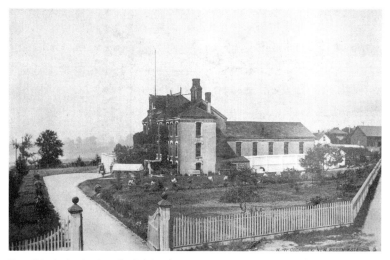

New Westminster Provincial Gaol. IMAGE A-03353 COURTESY OF ROYAL BC MUSEUM, BC ARCHIVES.

ately ill or injured people and brought them to the hospital. Many of these people were eking out a living in out-of-the-way places, some in primitive log cabins or even simple lean-tos, and it was only due to the Sisters' outreach program that some of them were saved. They found one fifty-two-year-old Irishman, entered in the records only as "Mr. Murphy," in an isolated hut. His ailment is not recorded, but he was in desperate condition and grateful for the merciful appearance of the Sisters, who transported him by canoe over ten miles—probably the first water ambulance in BC. He was admitted to hospital on November 16, 1887. Before he died a few days later, he is reported to have said, "What have I done to merit that God should grant me a little bit of Heaven, even before entering the great eternal Heaven?" It appears the Sisters even paid the thirty-five dollars for Mr. Murphy's funeral.

At a time when the few nurses working in hospitals were actually male orderlies, the Sisters ignored every social convention about where a proper woman could be found or with whom. They visited every door in those early years, including those of the jails and prisons, notorious for their poor sanitary conditions. Three of their first jail visits were to men who had been condemned to hang. Their primary commitment to compassionate care took them into every corner of human society, even among murderers and the tormented, screaming "lunatics" locked up in jails because there was no other place for them. The Sisters' willingness to freely interact with sufferers, to care for those in neglected conditions, and to provide the cleaning of wounds and injuries to prevent infection was intended to provide healing to the spirit as well as the body.

5

Fire and Epidemic, 1887–1919

IN THE EARLY DAYS OF SAINT MARY'S EXISTENCE, its financial situation was always precarious because the hospital carried a large debt and the Sisters stubbornly refused to allow financial considerations to cause anyone to go without care. In fact, in the first two years so many indigents were taken in that the Sisters could not pay operational expenses. Their solution to this problem was to widen their fundraising efforts. It was now proposed that there be no place off limits and that they should set out to canvass the roughest, most violent, most dangerous mining camps for money, and in 1888 Sister Leocadie and Sister Ethelbert made their first trip to the Cariboo mines. While the gold rush had peaked in 1865, the area still had a large population because the original claims were still being reworked and new riches were being discovered; in fact, the Cariboo would continue to produce for another fifty years. Thus, by the time the Sisters set out, the population of the camps had become a little more stable, which meant that they were more likely to find accommodation.

People in polite society, however, still considered women who turned up in the mining camps to be nothing more than prostitutes, so they were aghast at the idea of the Sisters riding out on horses, sleeping at night near the men in the camps or, even more incredibly, in the very same cabins—on one trip the Sisters lived for ten days in a cabin with several miners and CPR workers—and travelling unprotected with large sums of money. But while genteel society found the Sisters' willingness to go out and beg for help in these rough surroundings surprising, the miners themselves were even more surprised. Imagine the rough miner, seeking his fortune and spending it mostly on booze and other indulgences, being greeted by a nun on horseback asking for a donation for the Catholic hospital in New Westminster. As well, some of the Sisters spoke only French and could only ask for donations in broken English, but this was not always such a great disadvantage since the miner himself might well speak only German or Chinese.

The Sisters returned from that first trip with the large sum of $2,150, and this success encouraged them to make these arduous begging tours once or twice a year after that. Sometimes they were accompanied by a priest for protection, although often the priest was more nervous than the Sisters amid the rough and tumble of the work camps. They travelled not only in the warm spring and summer months amid abundant swarming mosquito populations but also in the late fall when it was difficult to find dry shelter from British Columbia's long rains, and even undertook their tours in the harsher conditions of winter. In one camp, the cabin they sheltered in was heated by a stove made of cans—an empty kerosene can on top of four empty oyster cans.

On one occasion they faced a hungry pack of wolves, on another an angry grizzly. A large tent fire roared through one camp they were canvassing, while some of the First Nations people they encountered were still engaged in local warfare and raiding and suspicious of the Sisters' intentions. Some of their tours exposed the Sisters to the dangerous working conditions that brought people to their hospital. Once, when an explosion shook the hut they were staying in and brought down a storm of debris, the startled Sisters were certain they were going to die, but they had just survived the use of dynamite by miners working a few feet away. It is probably fortunate that they were inside the hut at the time.

The Sisters' fundraising drives were not, however, limited to their Cariboo tours. They were diligent in visiting every little town and business, and where twenty dollars might be collected in some small hamlet, a business donation might be all of ten dollars. However, on the whole, Saint Mary's Hospital was kept alive by money from working men—the miners of the Cariboo, the fishermen and cannery workers on the Fraser River, the loggers in the bush and the railroaders on the line. Men like the twenty-eight-year-old Scottish brakeman T. Binnie and the twenty-eight-year-old Irish conductor John Fraser, whose injuries were taken care of by the Sisters at Saint Mary's, knew how much they needed hospitals, and they showed they were willing to pay to keep Saint Mary's going with their donations. As a result, most of the $1,500 to $3,000 the Sisters raised each year through donations came from them.

In 1889 the Royal Columbian Hospital, which had been

situated less than a block away from Saint Mary's, moved to new facilities in Sapperton, a move some said was politically motivated. This left Saint Mary's as the primary hospital serving the centre and west side of town and the industrial area along the river. To help with the added workload, they now employed five servants, but when the hospital had too many patients for even the Sisters and their servants to take care of—as happened in the typhoid epidemic between July 1890 and July 1891—the Sisters gave up their begging tours instead of giving up their visits to the sick, even though at this time the hospital was $20,000 in debt.

Within a few years, however, a long and hard economic depression hit the province and thousands were thrown out of work; fewer workers meant fewer injuries and therefore fewer patients for Saint Mary's. As the economic situation worsened, the Sisters increased their visits to people in their homes. The *Chronicles of Saint Mary's Hospital* state that between 1892 and 1897, although some patients still came to the hospital, it was far more likely that the hospital would go to them; in 1892 alone the seven Sisters on staff made some six hundred visits to the sick in their homes. They also served far more meals to the poor. These meals were provided both because this was a natural part of the Sisters' calling to care for the body and the spirit and because they understood the importance of good nutrition to prevent illness. In fact, Catholic nursing Sisters had insisted on good nutrition to aid in patient recovery as far back as the Middle Ages, long before mainstream medicine recognized its importance.

While the Sisters welcomed and celebrated a small number of conversions during these years, there is no evidence at any time to suggest that such conversions were sought from the unwilling. There were, of course, Bibles in the hospital and the Sisters had a chapel where they prayed twice each day, but their approach was to present Christianity to the patients and to practise their religion in a manner consistent with the rules of their order; there were no aggressive attempts to convert.

In 1891 typhoid became epidemic in New Westminster, ravaging the small city, and Saint Mary's histories proudly record how the hospital dealt with the epidemic with grace and determination, opening its doors to all, rich and poor. Typhoid had been initially carried into British Columbia about 1880, just a few years before Saint Mary's opened, by railway construction workers—an unexpected and unwelcome consequence of Confederation. From the start it was a difficult disease to combat because it can be contracted from asymptomatic patients, meaning that an infected person can give it to someone else before they exhibit symptoms. The bacteria that causes it, *Salmonella typhi*, can be carried by water, milk and food, especially fish and shellfish, and it is easily spread in crowded and unsanitary conditions. In British Columbia, where the fatality rate ranged anywhere from 3 to 7 percent in communities swept by the disease, a common response was to blame the Chinese and other workers on the railways. As a result, in some places Chinese labourers were forced to live on the outskirts of towns. Ironically, away from the polluted cities, they were safer than most of the population and thus typhoid was rare in their camps.

It is not clear how many people were admitted with typhoid fever to St Mary's Hospital in 1891 as some cases are clearly listed as typhoid while others were listed simply as "fever," but oral history tells of cots in the hallways and of the hospital's entry foyer overflowing with the ill. The patient intake increased from a norm of 250 per year to 300, even though for the most part only those in the worst condition sought help. Initially people brought to the hospital in the summer of 1891 were "indigents," and in the hospital's *Chronicles* one Sister reported that "the Sisters receive these with open heart, relying on Divine Providence for the payment of bills. With the care received and the severe diet they are made to follow, after a few weeks these patients are able to go back to their work."[31] But as they could not pay for their care, they placed a heavy load on a hospital that was already overburdened with debt.

Hospital histories often state that "none were lost who came to the hospital."[32] In fact, some people did die, among them labourers Mr. McMullen and Tom Franklin, twenty-four-year-old tailor James Rogers, eleven-year-old Ross Walter, and four-year-old Harry Wilcock. Still, remarkably few people admitted to Saint Mary's with typhoid did succumb, and the Sisters' strong ethic of cleanliness in the hospital, modern nursing techniques, and constant care without regard to their own safety likely had much to do with this fact. Meanwhile, outside the overflowing Saint Mary's, the typhoid epidemic caused deaths in New Westminster to increase in 1891 by 82 percent, up from 65 in 1890 to 118 in 1891 in a population of roughly 6,700. And along with the epidemic came real fear among those who weren't affected.

The effect of Saint Mary's success with typhoid patients was itself epidemic. Many people who had been reluctant to support a Catholic hospital were now won over. "They were not only cured from typhoid fever but cured of their prejudices."[33]

The community now gave Saint Mary's much stronger and unambiguous support, and extra donations were given to the hospital to help cover the costs of ministering to patients who could not afford to pay. That year marked the beginning of the City of New Westminster's annual donation toward the hospital's Christmas dinner, and the city fathers even decided to give back the $375 that had been collected from the hospital in taxes, a sum that was of great assistance at that time.

In the fall of 1895 Lady Aberdeen, the wife of Canada's Governor General, visited Saint Mary's Hospital. An ardent crusader for women's welfare and advancement at all levels of society, she was absolutely opposed to any class or religious distinctions, and shortly after her husband was appointed to his post in 1893 she set about establishing a branch of the International Council of Women in Canada and encouraging Canadian women to set up local councils that would bring together already existing women's organizations. In time they would become known as Canada's "Women's Parliament." Later Lady Aberdeen also became a driving force behind the organization of the Victorian Order of Nurses.

In 1891 she and Lord Aberdeen had bought the Coldstream Ranch near Vernon, so it was inevitable that they spent considerable time in BC and, because of Lady Aberdeen's interest in women's organizations, she was eager to tour institutions here run by women. Such places were very rare in Canada at that time, most of the significant ones being those belonging to religious orders, mostly Catholic nuns. On Lady Aberdeen's visit to Saint Mary's that fall she was welcomed by music played by a Native boys' band under the tutelage of the Oblate Brothers and with "the presentation of a bouquet to Lady Aberdeen by

Mr. Armstrong's granddaughter."[34] This was the most important recognition that the hospital had received, and for many years afterwards the publications of the National Council of Women would highlight the work being done there.

Charity hospitals are particularly vulnerable during times of depression, often left to operate with reduced government funding or no government support at all, as was the case for Saint Mary's between 1895 and 1897, the worst of the depression years. The hospital was hit particularly hard as the proportion of patients who could pay dropped significantly. Still, the Sisters continued to take in all patients without any hesitation, incurring more expenses along the way. Then, in typical fashion, they simply and optimistically celebrated the nature of their work in their *Chronicles*: "However, during these years the spiritual harvest is great, as many of these indigents who for years have neglected their God come back to Him in love and repentance."[35]

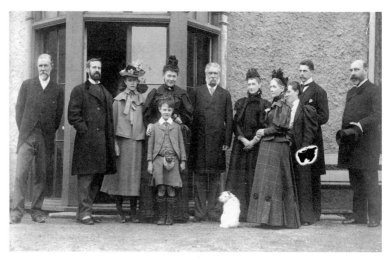

Lady Aberdeen, in centre behind child, during her 1895 visit. IMAGE A-01071
COURTESY OF ROYAL BC MUSEUM, BC ARCHIVES.

Fortunately for New Westminster and the hospital, in 1897 the city became a major stopping point for miners on the way to another gold rush, this time in the Klondike. When both patient numbers and donations began to increase, the Sisters, having successfully pulled their hospital through the tough times, proceeded with the construction of a new surgery. The cost was $2,923, and, to pay for it, Sisters Heloise and Praxedes set out on yet another canvassing tour. After six months on the road begging for contributions, they returned successful to New Westminster on November 4, 1897.

Although Catholic orders are not commonly thought of as women's rights organizations, some orders have a long history of caring for and advocating for women. This was especially true of the Sisters of Charity of Providence; the first work of its founder, Mother Emilie Gamelin, had been to open her large "yellow house" in Montreal to provide care and shelter for thirty elderly women. So in July 1898 when a Local Council of Women was formed in New Westminster to advance the interests of women, the Sisters of Providence at Saint Mary's became a driving force within it. Although the rules of their order did not allow the Sisters to represent the Council publicly or to hold office, they did attend the meetings and sought to have the Council take on issues of interest to them and provided key leadership for many of the Council's projects.

At the local Council's first meeting, likely in the old IOOF Hall, several of the Sisters met with a number of Protestant church women and others to hammer out a list of their priorities. Their position on suffrage was perfectly clear—they supported the Women's Franchise Bill. Of course, the Sisters of Saint Mary's Hospital and the other orders could not take a public position on the matter or sign petitions, but they participated in the discussions and planning at meetings. (Interestingly, the 1898 voters list shows only one voter living at Saint Mary's Hospital—George Cote, a steward. The nurses, the Sisters and even the hospital's superior, Sister Roderick, could not vote.) Since provincial legislation had already been passed allowing women to run for school boards—if they owned property—the Local Council of Women also made an attempt to recruit a Mrs. M.A. Kennedy of Sapperton to run for school board. Unfortunately, she declined as she feared the poor transportation between Sapperton and the rest of the city would prevent her from doing her duties should she be elected.

Health-care concerns were next on the Local Council's list, and here the expertise and assistance of the Sisters of Providence were invaluable. Back in 1887 when Saint Mary's had opened its doors, few women patients had been admitted because at that time most women gave birth at home. However, the death rate from birth complications was very high, particularly among women living in the countryside with no ready access to a doctor should things go wrong. As a result, women's organizations had begun to encourage safer birth procedures and healthier childcare, but initially they could not convince hospitals or government to take the issue seriously. In 1893 the Women's Christian Temperance Union (WCTU) had led a drive to establish an eight-bed maternity hospital, and it opened as Women's Hospital a year later at 212 3rd Avenue. As the Sisters of Saint Mary's were able to provide valuable practical medical assistance, they held a seat on the board of the new hospital. However, while this facility fulfilled a definite need in the community, the task of operating it quickly became overwhelming for the small group of women involved in its creation. This problem was resolved in 1898 when the Local Council of Women decided to make the success of Women's Hospital one of their priorities. They formed a hospital board from the member organizations of the council, and when the hospital was turned over to this board later that year, the Sisters of Providence again held a seat on it and found themselves not only running Saint Mary's but helping to run the maternity hospital.

In 1899, of the fifteen organizations making up the Local Council of Women, ten represented churches, and three of those were organizations of Catholic Sisters, including the Sisters of Providence of Saint Mary's Hospital. While this situation was fraught with opportunities for religious conflict, it was avoided through rules that were sensitive to differences. For example, the opening prayer at Council meetings was silent to prevent disputes over what form of prayer would be appropriate. And in order for the Catholic Sisters to participate without appearing to be involved in political activities, a system was devised for elections in which nominations to the executive were anonymous. Only the Council's secretary knew which group or member had nominated a candidate to stand for the executive, and elections were conducted by sealed ballot.

In 1900 the National Council of Women encouraged all local councils to establish branches of the Red Cross Society, and with Saint Mary's Hospital on its board this was promptly accomplished. The Local Council undertook child advocacy and pushed for a youth curfew in the city (city council resisted), and they campaigned for the creation of a kindergarten. They also called on government to do more regarding the "care of aged and infirm poor,"[36] a problem that the Sisters of Providence had recognized since they first came to the city. And in 1904 Dr. Charles Fagan, who had been Saint Mary's first medical director, worked with the Local Council of Women to form an association for the prevention of tuberculosis.

On Saturday, September 10, 1898, the Sisters of Providence at Saint Mary's Hospital, exhausted by coping with yet another outbreak of typhoid fever, were enjoying a well-deserved rest when they were awakened to the strangeness of a night sky lit up as if it were day. They could smell smoke in the air, but that wasn't unusual as the hot summer had led to numerous brush fires nearby and smoke had often drifted into the city. But looking out of their windows, they could see that there was a light coming from near the cathedral, and the Sisters who ventured outside felt a strong wind. Then fire gongs and bells began to ring out, waking the city.

Two hundred tons of hay had caught fire in Brackman and Ker's warehouse on the wharf, and from there it took only ten minutes for the fire to reach the brick buildings of Front Street. Then suddenly the entire downtown area of the city was ablaze. The city was "a sea of flames."[37] Meanwhile, another disaster was happening along the shore. The sternwheelers *Gladys*, *Edgar* and *Bon Accord*, all tied to the wharf, had caught fire, and when their mooring ropes burned through, they drifted downriver, setting all the warehouses and canneries aflame along their way. Soon the Sisters could see a line of flame extending from the foot of the hill below the hospital right across the entire waterfront. Firefighters tried to get close to the wharves but were soon pushed back to Columbia Street by the heat and the wind blowing the flames toward them. There, curious crowds had gathered on the street, with no idea that it was now just the other side of the buildings. Suddenly nearly all the buildings on the south side of the street burst into flame, and so intense had the fire already become that the windows across the street from them burst from the heat.

When the fire first broke out, a city alderman had been dispatched to open the fire gate to the city's water mains, which would have provided fire hydrants with high pressure for at least nine hours. But the alderman mistakenly tried to open a nearby gate instead of the water gate and, when the key wouldn't work, he left it there, too embarrassed to tell the firefighters who had sent him that he could not get it open. As a result, the firefighters were hampered by low water pressure while fighting the Lower Mainland's biggest fire in living memory.

Although onlookers still gathered to watch as Columbia Street and the waterfront burned, the noise of the fire made communication nearly impossible. More buildings began to catch fire, ignited by the heat alone. As the sparks from the fire landed on dry shingled roofs, thousands pulled their furniture and belongings out of their burning houses and fled. As explosions shook the ground and shattered glass fell onto the streets, those who were still inside buildings or fleeing up the hill were further endangered. The population of the city was in panic and tears. "The smoke, the crackling of the fire, the explosions, the wailing of the people are pathetic."[38] From Saint Mary's the Sisters watched as flames burned from every window of the six-storey Wintemute furniture factory at the corner of Fourth and Carnarvon streets. At last all they could see of the upper floors was pure fire, then the building was rocked by explosions and with a great roar it all fell inward in a massive collapse of brick and stone. (Just that past July, Mrs. J. Wintemute had been a patient at Saint Mary's Hospital, spending four days for an operation.)

As the fire burned through that night and the next day, the Sisters faced the prospect of losing the hospital. The city's water supply, including that in the hospital's own water tower, had been quickly depleted. Now the dry wooden building looked out over a fire that had pushed its way up the hill to a point just kitty-corner to it, and it was throwing out burning embers as large as small barrels. It was a true firestorm, and it was just outside. The Sisters hurried to evacuate the patients from the hospital and then brought out a small painting of the Madonna, which the superior, Sister Roderick, held out in front of the hospital for as long as she could withstand the heat, praying for

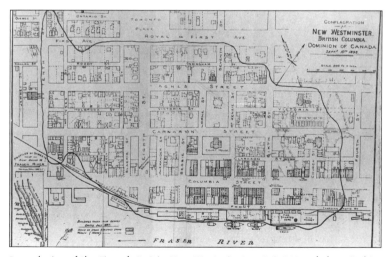

Boundaries of the Fire of 1898 in New Westminster. Saint Mary's hospital is just outside the fire zone at Fourth and Agnes streets in the upper right-hand corner of the map. Miraculously, the hospital was scorched but did not burn down in the fire and was able to take in patients and provide relief to the fire's victims. COURTESY OF NEW WESTMINSTER PUBLIC LIBRARY #1876.

the protection of Saint Mary. Three times she went out to face the flames holding the Madonna and three times was forced back inside by the unbearable heat, and yet courageously she went out again a fourth time, holding the painting and her faith out against the flames. And the fire did shift, leaving the buildings nearby in ashes but sparing Saint Mary's Hospital. For many years, that painting of the Madonna was kept in the hospital, although the bottom of the frame had been scorched by the heat of the flames that had failed to reach out far enough to set the hospital burning.

The buildings to the front and side of the hospital were gone, leaving a view of devastation from the windows of the hospital. Everything had vanished. The hotels, the wharves, the sternwheeler ships, the entire commercial district, the west end, Herring's Opera House, Saint Peter's Cathedral and the other churches, the CPR buildings, City Hall, even the Fire Hall— all destroyed. What was left was three inches of ash and dust. Here and there, burned sections of abandoned firehose lay on the streets between the ruins of a fallen city. The smoke of the fire had travelled upriver into the Fraser Valley and ash covered the shore in Surrey. Even after a few days there were wisps of smoke and small fires on the edge of the burned area. But the Sisters had refused to let their hospital go, faced the flames with prayer and faith, and now Saint Mary's miraculously remained to take in the injured and the refugees.

In the desperation and confusion some of the injured did not arrive at the hospital immediately. With all familiar landmarks wiped away, many experienced severe disorientation. Among those injured was the McGonigle family. Mrs. McGonigle had awakened to the sound of cracking windows and, looking from the windows of their living quarters at the back of their store on Front Street, she had seen the flames and realized that they were already completely surrounded by the fire. Wearing only nightclothes, she and her husband gathered their children and ran through the flames. The children's clothes caught fire, but the family struggled on to safety in their bare feet through the burning streets. Where they spent the next day is unknown, but on September 12 they were admitted to Saint Mary's Hospital. Mrs. P. McGonigle, aged thirty-three, her eight-year-old daughter May, six-year-old son James, and three-year-old daughter Florence all had badly burned feet and remained in the hospital until November. The family had lost everything and little Florence was permanently disabled. The entire family of storekeeper H.B. Grossman was also admitted

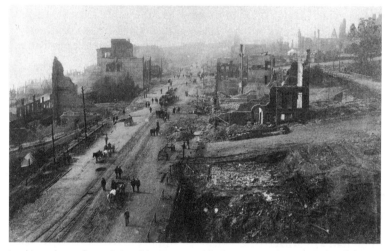

Looking down from Columbia Street, with the Fraser River outside of the photographed area to the left, taken from the top of the Burr Block the day after the fire. The haze in the photograph accurately displays the smoky conditions. Saint Mary's Hospital is just a few blocks up the hill from this location. PHOTOGRAPH COURTESY OF NEW WESTMINSTER PUBLIC LIBRARY #3123.

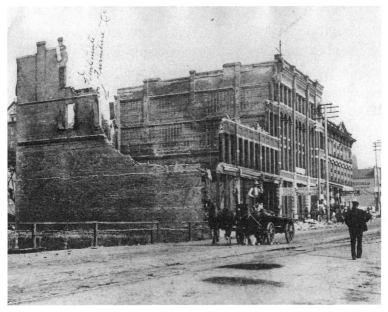

The Wintemute family's furniture store after the Great Fire. Both the Wintemute company store and factory burned to the ground. The family had lost their home to fire the previous August. PHOTOGRAPH COURTESY OF NEW WESTMINSTER PUBLIC LIBRARY #235.

to the hospital; among the five family members was their three-week-old baby.

The first relief in the form of tents for the five-hundred homeless families came from Vancouver by streetcar. The armoury became headquarters for relief, with much of the activity there under the direction of the women who just that summer had organized the Local Council of Women with Saint Mary's Hospital as a member. Meanwhile, fast action by Mayor Thomas Ovens and Provincial Secretary Fred J. Hume and the surrounding cities provided relief and helped to prevent hunger. (Ovens had himself been a patient at the hospital on more than one occasion and had just been admitted May 10 and released June 6 for a "surgical operation."[39])

In the immediate aftermath of the fire, Saint Mary's Hospital served 845 meals, gave out 300 prescriptions, and made 130 visits to treat out-patients injured by the fire. As well, the Sisters gave medical care to roughly 150 of the injured who came to the hospital's open doors. Fortunately, the benefactors who had been won over to support the hospital through the Sisters' valiant work in the typhoid epidemic of 1891, just eight years prior, now rushed to help. Alexander Ewen, a salmon-cannery owner, sent fish to help feed the hungry, a sawmill provided the hospital with firewood, and those merchants who still had stock that had not been burned provided the necessary fruit and vegetables.

The misery took some time to subside and kept Saint Mary's busy for weeks. Long after the flames were extinguished the smoke from the fire continued to cause suffering, and for many weeks there was a large increase in the number of patients admitted for sore throats and respiratory ailments. Then in the crowded conditions after the fire while the homeless received shelter wherever they could, there was another outbreak of typhoid. One of the city's schoolteachers, twenty-three-year-old W.E. McKenzie, had to leave his already traumatized students behind while he struggled in hospital with the disease for eleven days in early October. The effort to rebuild homes, businesses and the city was sometimes exhausting, as was demonstrated by the case of civil engineer J.R. Roy, aged twenty-five, admitted on September 19, eight days after the fire, for fatigue. Those who survived the fire would often be haunted by it. In their book, *The Great Fire of 1898*, Archie and Dale

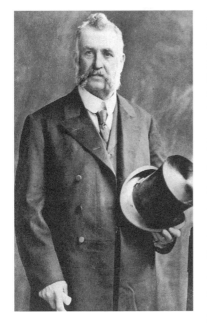

Thomas Ovens, Mayor of New Westminster during the Great Fire of 1898 and patient of Saint Mary's Hospital. PHOTO COURTESY OF NEW WESTMINSTER PUBLIC LIBRARY #581.

Miller tell of a woman who cried because there were no familiar buildings left for her to know where she was. And in December 1900, two years after the fire, fireman Paul McTaggart, aged twenty-six, was admitted to the hospital for more than a month for "melancholy." Ironically the Great Fire of 1898 improved local health when it burned out the older parts of the city, reducing communicable diseases.

Saint Mary's Hospital did receive some money from the relief fund, and it was recorded in the October receipts as "New Westminster Relief Fund for Patients sent from Fire $185."[40] That month, brandy sold to patients to soothe their pain earned the hospital another seven dollars, and in November another $126.25 came from the relief fund.

While the Great Fire of 1898 was more than enough for Saint Mary's to cope with, there was another calamity in the offing. On October 4, 1899, the Sisters of the Good Shepherd Convent and Orphanage burned down in just half an hour, leaving sixty-four people homeless, most of them children. With the city still rebuilding after the fire, there was literally no place for these newly homeless people to go. The Sisters of Saint Ann had only room to take in thirty of the children, and with a hospital already full of patients, the Sisters of Providence had no beds available. Instead, they gave up their dormitory, infirmary and community room to house the other thirty-four people, and moved their own mattresses to the attic.

The orphans from the fire at the Good Shepherd Orphanage were still living at the hospital while awaiting the completion of the new Providence Orphanage, when Saint Mary's Hospital was again asked to respond to an emergency. The sternwheeler *Ramona*, with Captain Charles Seymour in command, had departed New Westminster for Chilliwack on April 10, 1901, on a routine voyage with a large cargo and nineteen passengers. At Fort Langley the ship's aboriginal crew loaded a horse and wagon aboard for transport to the other side of the river. The ship crossed the river, the horse

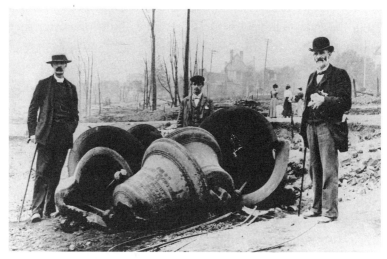

Cracked and broken bells of Holy Trinity Anglican Church, 1898. PHOTOGRAPH COURTESY OF NEW WESTMINSTER PUBLIC LIBRARY #268.

Receipt book of Saint Mary's Hospital for November 1898, shows a payment of $126.25 made to the hospital by the relief fund for the care of the injured after the Great Fire. COURTESY OF NEW WESTMINSTER MUSEUM AND ARCHIVES MANUSCRIPT #302.

and wagon were unloaded, and the ship turned upriver again. It was at this point that passenger Mrs. Hector Morrison and another woman, unlike most of the passengers who were enjoying the scenery and weather from the upper deck, decided to go below to chat with the ship's crew. Not long after they went below on this fine April day the passengers on the upper deck felt and heard a huge explosion.

The explanation for the explosion dated back to 1898 when the Lower Fraser River Navigation Company, which owned the *Ramona*, had put the ship on the New Westminster to Ladner route in direct competition with the ship *Transfer*. The rivalry had become intense, and the two ships often raced on the river, but as victory usually went to the *Transfer*, the *Ramona's* owners had refitted the ship with a new high-pressure boiler. And it was this boiler that had exploded. In his book, *Shipwrecks of British Columbia*, Fred Rogers gives this account by a passenger on board the *Ramona* that day:

The explosion first sounded like a dull rumble, then the ship heaved up and shook violently. After the steam and smoke cleared, about six persons were in the water and someone tried to throw life rings to them. The ship still had headway and passed by for a short distance, leaving them behind so that the life rings were of no use. Some men were trying to launch a lifeboat, but in the confusion it flooded and was useless. Another boat was lowered and this one floated. There was a great deal of screaming and noise from below. The captain had a hard time to restore order but he soon got the men fighting the fires. He was very concerned about the flames reaching the hay, kerosene, and explosives that were stowed with the freight.[41]

When the smoke cleared, it was discovered that Mrs. Morrison and her companion were floating dead in the water, several

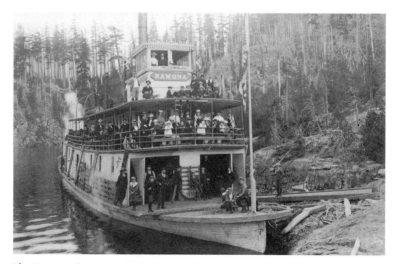

The *Ramona* in 1904. PHOTOGRAPH BY W.T. COOKSLEY, COURTESY OF NEW WESTMINSTER PUBLIC LIBRARY #2376.

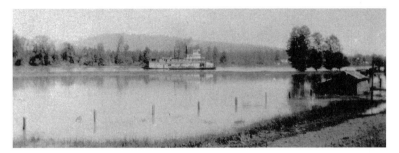

The *Ramona* on the Fraser River. IMAGE C-09117 COURTESY OF ROYAL BC MUSEUM, BC ARCHIVES.

other passengers and crewmen were struggling to avoid drowning, and a Native crewman was badly injured, with blood streaming down his face. Though a bucket brigade was quickly started to douse the flames, with the boilers gone, the *Ramona* was now adrift and in danger of going aground. The situation was brought under control when someone with a level head dropped the anchors, the bodies of the women were pulled from the river and rescues were made.

The injured crew and passengers of the *Ramona* were brought to Saint Mary's Hospital. Many of them had severe burns so they had long stays in the hospital, and some did not survive. Since outpatients were not listed in the hospital records, however, it is not known how many of the survivors in total were treated there.

By 1902 the Sisters had again become frustrated with the lack of support and funding from the provincial government, but they noted in their *Chronicles* that the City of New Westminster had, on the other hand, responded to the lack of provincial support by providing free water, while Ewen's fish cannery continued to provide unlimited supplies of fish and a local sawmill donated firewood. Over the years this lack of support or even interest on the part of the provincial government would continue to stand in stark contrast to the strength of support in the community served by and most familiar with the hospital. The nature of this relationship between the hospital and the community was amply demonstrated from 1902 to 1904 when the New Westminster Bridge was constructed across the Fraser River. As the construction site was just down the hill from Saint Mary's, the contractor organized a health-insurance plan with the Sisters of Providence. Each bridge employee was charged one dollar a month for health care, with two-thirds going to the doctor and one-third going to Saint Mary's.

Although bridge construction was considered the most dangerous of all work at this time, there were only two fatalities on the New Westminster Bridge, a fact that led to its being known for many years as "The Lucky Bridge." However, many

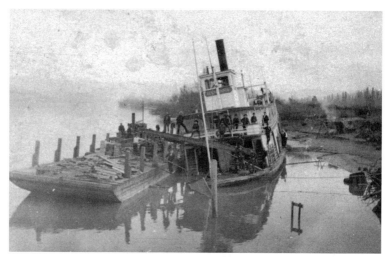

The *Ramona* beached at McKay's Landing. IMAGE C-09086 COURTESY OF ROYAL BC MUSEUM, BC ARCHIVES.

of the bridge workers did make use of their Saint Mary's health-insurance plan. There are numerous notations in the hospital register of 1902 to 1904 of labourers with broken bones, which may or may not have been related to bridge work, but some patients are specifically recorded as being bridge builders. One of these was Robert Balfour, the main contractor for substructure and approaches to the bridge. A civil engineer, he had come west from Ontario as a bridge inspector for the CPR and in 1886 had been elected to Vancouver's first city council.

Although the bridge was built for trains and wheeled traffic, it seems to have also brought a different sort of traffic into the city. In the years that it was under construction, there are a number of women recorded in Saint Mary's patient register as prostitutes, though none were recorded before this time. And when the bridge was completed, the patient register strangely and suddenly stops recording prostitutes. In general throughout Saint Mary's history prostitutes and persons with syphilis were the two categories of patients most likely to go to another hospital rather than seek care from the Sisters, but it is possible that, given the excellent care that the bridge workers were receiving, the women with whom they associated also went to Saint Mary's for help.

The bridge opened on July 23, 1904, and the occasion was marked by a night of torchlight dancing on the bridge by Chehalis Natives, fireworks and a lighted procession of ships. For the Sisters, nurses and staff of Saint Mary's Hospital it was time to say goodbye to the bridge workers they had tended, visited and watched over for three years. However, the hospital directly benefited from the new bridge again in 1910 when the BC Electric Railway's morning milk train began crossing the bridge from Surrey to New Westminster, allowing easier access to large quantities of fresh milk. (New Westminster Bridge can still be seen today as the railway bridge that runs below the Pattullo Bridge.)

Even while the bridge was under construction, the work of the hospital had continued in treating and controlling diseases that tended to break out mainly in the poorest areas of the city, and in 1903 and 1904 an unknown ailment resulted in large numbers of sick children being admitted to hospital. Soon several of the nurses had also fallen ill and became patients as well. The incident underlined the dangers but also the dedication of a hospital that would refuse to see the poor waste away alone in the city's shacks behind quarantine signs or left to die in the streets.

On October 2, 1905, British Columbia's Lieutenant-Governor, Henri-Gustave Joly de Lotbinière, visited the hospital. De Lotbinière had sat in the Quebec Assembly from 1867 to 1885 and had even served very briefly as that province's premier. In 1896 he had joined Prime Minister Laurier's government as controller (later minister) of Inland Revenue and was rewarded for his service by being made BC's Lieutenant-Governor in 1900. Although not popular among the English-speaking people of this province, he took a great interest in those from Quebec, especially the French-speaking Sisters of Providence.

The year 1905 continued to see a strong relationship between the hospital and the local community. The city council increased its donation for Saint Mary's annual Christmas dinner to fifty dollars and Mayor W.H. Keary personally donated another twenty dollars. It was also the year that the first formal organization of lay women assisting the hospital was formed, the Catholic Women of New Westminster, and the Sisters of Providence took this opportunity to hand over their role on the Local Council of Women to the new group and move into the background. Women's Hospital, one of their primary concerns, had been absorbed by the Royal Columbian two years earlier after unsuccessfully seeking the same government funding as went to other hospitals. While the loss of Women's Hospital had been the start of the Royal Columbian's maternity ward, as more and more women chose to give birth in hospital, many of them began to choose Saint Mary's and the little hospital added maternity to the already long list of its important roles in the community.

The next few years saw Saint Mary's fall on hard times as a new economic recession struck, once again wiping out its established role as the hospital for injured working men. Patient admissions slowly declined until in November 1910 not one person's name was entered in the register. With just six long-term patients, plus two elderly men and three elderly women to care for, Saint Mary's seemed to have outlived its usefulness, and the Mother House in Montreal made the decision to close it. At this point Dr. F. Kenny stepped in and bought the hospital time by convincing local authorities to support its conversion to an old folks home. The Mother House agreed and the hospital was spared, but the idea of an old folks home was never implemented because the local Archbishop refused to co-operate with the change. According to the *Chronicles*, "The Sisters continue to live from day to day, always on the verge of destitution yet never lacking anything."[42] Then, as the Sisters continued on, the patient numbers began to slowly increase again until in 1912 all of those seeking admittance could not be accommodated, and it became necessary to build a new wing on the hospital. The new space was twenty-seven feet by forty-six feet (some sources say thirty-seven feet by forty-six feet) and had room for twelve beds, a surgery, a pharmacy, a dressing room and a furnace. But the most important addition was that very modern convenience—a hand-operated, rope-and-pulley elevator! Prior to this time, nurses had to assist patients up the stairs to the second floor rooms; the third floor of the three-storey building had been used as the Sisters' quarters so that patients would not have to climb that extra flight of stairs.

In the spring of 1913 the special place in the community that Saint Mary's held was verified by the first recorded visit of the city's May Queen. Her entourage included Judge Frederic W. Howay of the County Court in New Westminster and city councillors Cambridge, Gilley and Lynch. A fine lunch was prepared for these guests before they were taken on a tour of

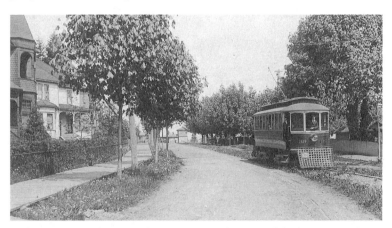

Park Row, across the street from Saint Mary's Hospital, looking toward Queen's Park. Circa 1910. By this time patients and visitors could come to the hospital by streetcar. JAIMIE McEVOY PRIVATE COLLECTION.

the hospital. Until it closed 90 years later, Saint Mary's was included in the May Queen's annual tour of the city's institutions, and with all of its fuss and ceremony and tea and ice cream it significantly encouraged the morale of the young children who were patients there, as well as the Sisters of Providence and the nursing staff.

In 1915 the Saint Mary's Hospital Society was established by laywomen whose purpose was to assist the hospital in any way necessary. As part of the Local Council of Women, they were active on health-care issues in both the hospital and community, campaigning successfully to have milk delivered in bottles rather than in cans, to have city garbage trucks covered, and to organize Better Babies contests to teach new mothers how to care for the health and nutrition of their infants. Dur-

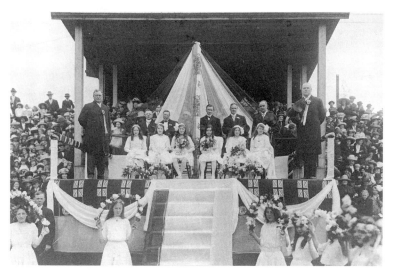

The first May Queen to start the annual visit to Saint Mary's Hospital was Jean McPhail in 1913. The hospital often involved children in the care and encouragement of other children who were patients at the hospital.
PHOTOGRAPH COURTESY OF NEW WESTMINSTER PUBLIC LIBRARY #3198.

ing World War I, Mrs. Lewis, president of the Hospital Society, also took over the representation of Saint Mary's on the Local Council of Women, making regular reports between the two organizations.

It is worth noting that by 1913 donations had started coming in from non-Catholic clubs as well,[43] and over the coming years the Elks, Scouts, Royal Canadian Legion and others raised money for the hospital. In 1916 New Westminster City Council, never on the sidelines when it came to health care, approved an additional grant of $350, and a year later the hospital, now thirty years old, began to benefit from the estates of former patients. The first came in October of that year when the hospital received property in the city's downtown area valued at $1,500 from the estate of the late Joseph Wise.

Meanwhile, provincial government funding in the form of a grant of five hundred dollars had only come for the first time in 1915. This elicited the closest thing to a sign of irritation or a negative thought ever expressed on record by the Sisters of Providence. They were totally frustrated with a government that had delayed funding for so many years and then, when it was provided, gave less than was given to other hospitals in British Columbia. But as this problem persisted, the Sisters themselves became more persistent. According to the *Chronicles of the Sisters of Providence*, on July 6, 1916, Sister M. Vincent, superior, sent two Sisters to Victoria to interview the Premier regarding fair compensation. "For many years past the Sisters have applied to the Provincial Government for financial assistance to care for the indigents who came seeking help," the *Chronicles* state, "but as the Royal Columbian Hospital is paid for the caring of the poor patients, Saint Mary's application was always rejected. . . . This benevolent man receives the Sisters most graciously and obtains for them five hundred dollars with the assurance that the same amount would be given the following year. The Mayor of New Westminster is also interviewed with the result that the City Council voted the sum of $350 for the relief of the suffering poor at Saint Mary's."[44] While over the years provincial politicians would come to see the insistent and idealistic Sisters as a problem, others occasionally saw that the excellent quality and breadth of the work at their hospital filled a real need and was deserving of support. "These amounts are greatly appreciated not so much for the money as for the idea that after years of asking, the Civic Authorities have at last recognized the good work that the Sisters of Saint Mary's are doing."[45]

When the church bells rang on November 11, 1918, everyone knew what it meant. The Great War was finally over! But it was a particularly sad day at Saint Mary's Hospital. As the celebration spread into the streets, the revellers passed the funeral procession for the city's latest influenza victim, Sister Joseph Napoleon, a thirty-year-old nurse who had served at Saint Mary's for three and a half years.

Understanding the role of Saint Mary's Hospital in the Spanish influenza epidemic of 1918–19 requires an understanding of the impact of the epidemic on the entire community. By the time World War I ended, 60,000 Canadians lay dead on the battlefields, and the signing of the armistice on November 11, 1918, brought a great sigh of relief in this country; there would be no more war dead. But many of the soldiers who had survived the fighting never made it back to Canada because they succumbed to Spanish influenza. They included men like Alan McCleod, who had won the Victoria Cross after shooting down three of the eight enemy aircraft that had attacked his plane. He lived through the crash of his plane in No Man's Land only to be killed by influenza. Colonel John McCrae, the surgeon and poet who wrote the poem "In Flanders Fields," also died of the disease. Lieutenant Charles Duncan of the 10th New Westminster Regiment, never even got overseas before he contracted influenza and died.

Then, as the soldiers who had fought to defend Canada came home again, they unwittingly brought this deadly killer back to their families and communities. In October 1918 every ship in one convoy bringing troops home had its flag at half-mast, and two of the ships, manned by crews ill with flu, collided at sea. The virus found its way to the West Coast as soldiers crossed the country by train, though it was not until November that the connection between the soldiers and the spread of the disease was realized. Then officials in more than forty towns imposed quarantines and closed their train stations.

Spanish influenza started like any other flu but developed into a quick and savage pneumonia. Patients' temperatures climbed to a burning 104 degrees F, delirium and severe dehydration left them exhausted, but despite their fevers they would complain of being freezing cold. Since antibiotics did not exist as yet and even aspirin in pill form was new and its use not at all widespread, sufferers tried old family and folk remedies like hot mustard plasters and cold compresses and herbal teas. One Vancouver doctor recommended patients put sulfur in their shoes. Another told his patients to eat yeast cakes. Weak vaccines that were invented to combat the plague were more likely to produce an infection than a cure. Mortality rates once

The death certificate of Sister Joseph Napoleon, also known as Florentine Aubin, nursing Sister at Saint Mary's Hospital who lost her life while caring for her patients. Buried on Armistice Day, November 11, 1918. IMAGE B-13091 COURTESY OF ROYAL BC MUSEUM, BC ARCHIVES.

the pneumonia set in reached 40 percent, but those who survived were so weak that they faced a long convalescence.

What was particularly odd about Spanish influenza was that, unlike other epidemics, it seemed to be most lethal among twenty- to forty-year-olds and, unfortunately, when it struck, the Lower Mainland was booming with ship construction and other industries related to the war effort. As a result, there were large numbers of men in that age bracket working in close quarters in the factories and living tightly packed in rooming houses, often sharing washrooms. Adding to the problem as Christmas approached were the hordes of men coming in by boat from remote logging camps; many were already ill as they arrived, some had died en route. These conditions increased the spread of infection.

The hospitals in the Lower Mainland, already busy with the increased population, had little excess capacity. Although there were debates in Parliament on the need for a national health body to deal with situations such as killer epidemics and to co-ordinate health care across the country, Canadian cities were actually left on their own to combat the flu. In New West-minster, with a population of 14,000, the third largest city in the province after Vancouver and Victoria, Dr. S.C. McEwan was in charge and, ignoring the debate in Vancouver that was delaying closures there, he closed all places of entertainment after just fifty cases had been confirmed and two flu deaths had occurred. Restaurants were allowed to stay open if they washed their dishes well and if they could get the customers to come, but diners were expected to eat quickly and then leave. Hotels and rooming houses in the city were inspected to ensure that precautions were being taken.

The impact of the flu on daily life was incredible. In October and November 1918 as quarantine signs became commonplace on houses throughout the city, all gatherings, private and public, in New Westminster were banned. Schools were closed. Pool halls and theatres were ordered closed. (In-terestingly, libraries recorded record numbers of book loans as people prepared to hunker down in their homes.) Union meetings were cancelled. Public weddings were put on hold. Even church congregations were forbidden to meet, which led to an altercation between the police and the Salvation Army, which had assembled for an outdoor meeting. Initially they refused to disperse, and it actually looked like a riot between the Salvation Army and the police might ensue, but cooler heads prevailed in the end. The police acknowledged that the Salvation Army had attempted to respect the ban on public meetings by meeting outdoors and conceded that the regulations were confusing; the Salvation Army in turn agreed to disperse without further incident.

Funeral processions still took place, and in New Westminster for the first time in its history they became an almost daily event. In the year 1918 the death rate increased in the little city by 47 percent with a total of 358 deaths, 116 more than in the previous year. Some 3 to 4 percent of the city's population died that year, at a time when Canadian death rates averaged only 1 percent of the population. The disease struck hardest in the fall of 1918 but would linger through much of the following year.

The police and fire departments had so many ill that they had trouble attending to regular duties. The Retail Clerks Association called for earlier closing times because those staff members remaining on the job were so exhausted from taking on the work of sick colleagues. "Closed because of flu" was a common sign on businesses. Ambulance drivers worked around the clock but the work became dangerous as some delirious patients were violent. So many letter carriers were ill that the mail couldn't be delivered on a daily basis any more, and since every telephone call had to be connected manually by an operator in those days and so many of them were sick, telephone customers were asked to limit their calls. With no one to harvest them, potatoes and other crops rotted in fields, although later in the epidemic, unions organized a temporary employment system for the Lower Mainland to help relieve farm labour shortages.

During the epidemic the great emphasis that was placed on personal hygiene, cleaning, disinfecting and hand washing would permanently change society's approach to cleanliness and health. But as stronger cleaning products grew scarce, the price of lemons shot through the roof, and "lemon clean" became a new hallmark of cleanliness. At Saint Mary's the nurses wrapped themselves in special white gowns in an effort to provide some protection, making them look like ghosts as they moved among patients in the low light at night. Wards were filled with extra beds placed almost next to each other so those struggling to survive were not spared the sight and sounds of those who were suffering and dying. The Sisters, however, hung sheets between the beds in an effort to minimize the effects of coughing and sneezing, a forerunner to the modern hospital bed curtain.

Many of the patients were children as Saint Mary's had taken in the sick from the Providence Orphanage when the flu spread among them, just as they had taken them in when the Good Shepherd Convent had burned in October 1899. Soon the wards were filled with crying and desperately ill children, and the doctors and nurses responded by working sixteen-hour shifts, going without sleep in an effort to comfort and save the lives of their charges. When even that was not enough to cope with the emergency, the Sisters recruited volunteer women who worked eight-hour shifts around the clock, taking over as nurses fell ill. Many of them were teachers whose schools had been

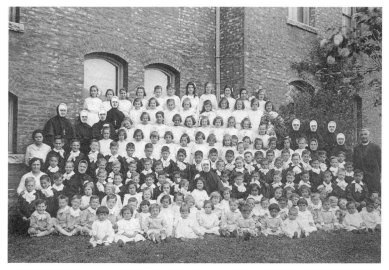

Providence Orphanage, June 16, 1918. While other schoolchildren had their schools closed and were sent home for safety, children in orphanages were still in close proximity to each other in large groups, despite the risk of infection, as the orphanage was their only home. Providence Orphanage was particularly hard hit by Spanish influenza, and many of the children in this photo had to be taken into Saint Mary's Hospital.
PHOTOGRAPH COURTESY OF OBLATE ARCHIVES, VANCOUVER, OBLATES OF MARY IMMACULATE (OMI), SAINT PAUL'S PROVINCE.

closed, so for some students the woman who had taught them just days before was now nursing them. Some teachers never returned to the classroom, succumbing to influenza themselves and giving their lives as volunteer nurses.

As hospital supplies ran out, volunteers collected sheets and blankets from the community, came forward to do the extra laundry and took food and medicine to houses under quarantine. One particular difficulty they encountered at quarantined homes was that often everyone in the family was too sick to keep the furnace stoked or to keep coal burning in the fireplaces. Some of these people died simply because there was no one to care for them. Throughout the province whole families and even a group of railway workers were found suffering from the flu and unable to fend for themselves and were rushed into whatever hospital space could be found for them. At the cemeteries, extra gravediggers had to be recruited to keep up with the burials. Roughly 4,400 British Columbians are estimated to have died from the deadly virus, about 1 percent of the province's population.

Doctor John Barker would remember, "I was still in bed when the armistice was signed. I remember the funerals passing along Sixth Avenue that same day. Nurses were almost unobtainable and doctors were so overworked that, during the time I was ill, I had five different doctors. They worked themselves into a state of exhaustion but returned as soon as possible when another one dropped. It was terrible. Many of my friends died."[46] It was estimated that two hundred doctors died while combatting influenza across Canada.

Roughly one in four nurses is estimated to have caught the disease because they were often already exhausted and in no condition to fight it off. In British Columbia, at least seventeen Sisters and nurses, some of them still students, died. The Registered Nurses Association of BC and others have called for a significant memorial to their sacrifice. While here and there some of them are remembered and honoured, no significant effort has been made to identify the names of all the doctors and nurses, professionals and volunteers, who gave their lives in the epidemic for the compassionate care of others and to honour them with a suitable memorial.

6

The Middle Years 1920–1956

THE ROARING TWENTIES BEGAN with Saint Mary's Hospital still working at full capacity to serve the community's needs. Typical of those who owed gratitude to the Sisters in these years was an Anglican family named Stokes, who lived across the street from the hospital. This is their story as told by Poppy (Stokes) Whitemore, aged eighty-eight, on August 11, 2005:

My family lived at 212 Agnes Street, across the street from Saint Mary's Hospital. I was born in Ireland on December 28, 1916. My father was from England and my mother had taught in Belfast. They met in Manitoba, though she lived in Saskatoon, and they married. Their last name was Stokes. I was born in Ireland because my mother went back there when my father fought in World War I.

I had the measles when I was four and had to be

quarantined, but I was also developing a mastoid in my ear and the doctor felt I should be hospitalized and under constant care. They did not have a room for me at Saint Mary's to keep me in isolation from the other patients so they let me stay in the nursing Sisters' quarters. We got to know the Sisters well, even though we were Anglican and attending Holy Trinity.

In 1924 when I was about seven years old, there was a fire at our house. It had four bedrooms, two to each side, with a patio at the front, and one night we were awakened with banging on the door. The back of the house was on fire. My father had a Model T Ford, and in those days you could unscrew the gas tanks. Someone had tried to steal the gas, and they held a match up to the gas tank to see if there was any gas inside. The gas tank had gas all right and it exploded!

The Sister nurses were all there, and they were distraught. They knew us well and thought we had all been killed. The house had transoms, those windows above the doors. Because my godmother was deaf, Dad had to get a stepladder while the house was on fire, and climb in through the transom to get her to safety. We kids were taken in and put up to live for a while in the hospital.

Afterwards our family moved a few blocks away. Saint Mary's got its milk from Booth's dairy across the bridge. Booth delivered his milk in a touring Ford motorcar and I remember he loved to whistle—he whistled all the time. So Booth left our milk at Saint Mary's (after the fire) and we would go there every day to get it.

My Mother died at Saint Mary's and I had two sons

born there. Eventually, Saint Mary's closed down, which was a bloody crime.

Regular annual funding from the provincial government for Saint Mary's had finally come in April 1923 in the amount of $590.05, equal to approximately 50 cents a day per patient. In return, the Sisters had to agree to allow government officials to visit and examine the books whenever they pleased; it was the first step toward the hospital's eventual complete integration into the public health-care system. By June of that year the government was also using taxes on liquor to provide money for hospitals, paying it out on the basis of twenty-five cents a day per patient; this came to $1,984 for Saint Mary's. It seemed that, at long last, Saint Mary's and the people it served would no longer be bypassed and ignored while other hospitals were supported, but as a result of this new funding, the hospital would gradually become reliant on the government and lose its independent sources of revenue.

But 1923 was also a year of loss. Saint Mary's beloved medical director, Dr. Richard Eden Walker, died at age fifty-nine on August 27. He had shared a partnership with Saint Mary's first medical director, Dr. Charles Fagan, and had served as president of the BC Medical Association in 1901–02 and held that post again at the time of his death. The Sisters had regarded him as particularly unselfish because of his willingness to treat those in need, and he had played a key role in helping to keep the hospital modern and up to date. He was succeeded by Dr. W.A. Clarke, who took over his practice and continued to provide support to the hospital.

The 1920s would see the installation of an automatic

elevator to replace the old rope-and-pulley one, cement sidewalks, oil heating and a coat of stucco for the hospital. In 1928 a nurses' home was built as, for the most part, nurses were expected to live in or near the hospital in which they served. The new home provided modern utilities and private rooms on the first floor for the ten lay nurses and on the second for the Sisters. In May of the following year, Dr. Clarke's mother, Mrs. R.E. Clarke, donated a new X-ray unit along with a bond of one thousand dollars.

In 1926 the hospital had begun to give out cash payments to some of the poor, implementing an early form of welfare. The statistics for December 31, 1926, show 1,615 meals for the poor, 507 prescriptions, but also $588.75 in cash allowances. Three years later the amount of these allowances to the poor had increased to $1,955.86, mostly to pay for clothing. And that same year a total of 2,107 meals was given out. Although officially the Great Depression had not begun, the rolls of the unemployed had been swelling steadily since the end of the war, and while Saint Mary's had never set itself up to serve meals to the poor, the Sisters had always simply given food to anyone who came knocking on the door. However, as the tough times became worse, long lines of the unemployed formed outside the hospital every mealtime. Native people were particularly hard hit during these years because, even after relief payments were introduced by the federal government in 1931, Native families received just five dollars instead of the fifteen dollars a month given to non-Natives because it was assumed that Native people could live off the land. But once again Saint Mary's gave care to all who were sick and provided meals for all who were hungry. In 1929 the numbers of poor seeking relief from hunger climbed above two thousand, and in 1931 and again in 1932 the Sisters served an incredible 5,500 meals. As in past emergencies, the community rallied behind the Sisters, with women volunteers supplying the hospital with about two hundred jars of fruit a year.

The early years of the Great Depression were, however, unusually good in a financial sense to Saint Mary's as money arrived providentially from estates. A Mrs. McNeilly left the hospital the extraordinarily large amount of $10,000, which in better times would have been enough to take care of Saint Mary's poor for the next five to ten years. And a Mr. Cassidy— perhaps the same Cassidy who had been the very first patient, a man too poor to be able to pay—willed the hospital $4,500.

Fortunately for New Westminster, Fred Hume, who was

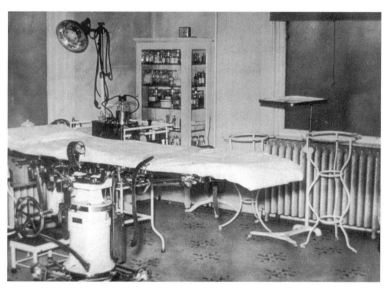

Operating room at Saint Mary's Hospital, circa 1935. Note the straps to hold down the patient. PHOTOGRAPH COURTESY OF NEW WESTMINSTER PUBLIC LIBRARY #2889.

mayor of the city from 1934 to 1942, sought to preserve and assist the city's institutions that were affected by the Depression. Although some, such as Columbian College, the oldest college in British Columbia, closed their doors forever, the mayor was able to arrange direct funding to Saint Mary's at the rate of fifty cents per day per patient and provided two men from the city's "relief" rolls as hospital employees, paid for by the city. The city's cheque to the hospital for 1936 amounted to $3,000, which was equivalent to six thousand days of medical care to the poor at the height of this difficult period. But at the same time the hospital was so overcrowded and the Sisters so overworked that, when its fiftieth anniversary arrived on July 1, 1936, they were too tired to organize celebrations.

The Depression was hard on doctors because even those whose practices had catered in the past to the upper and middle classes now found themselves with indigent patients, many of them prosperous people who had lost everything. With few people able to pay their doctors' fees, the doctors became as poor as their patients. The Sisters of Providence, seeking to rally and encourage the city's doctors to give aid to everyone in need, held a banquet for all of the doctors in New Westminster on the occasion of the installation of an X-ray machine on April 26, 1934.

Nurses also suffered during the Depression, and a Canadian government report in 1932 revealed that 40 percent of all nurses were unemployed. Eleven nursing schools across the country were forced to close. Ernest E. Winch and his son, Harold Winch, of the Canadian Co-operative Commonwealth Federation (CCF)—the longest serving father-and-son team in Canadian political history—were unsuccessful in their attempts

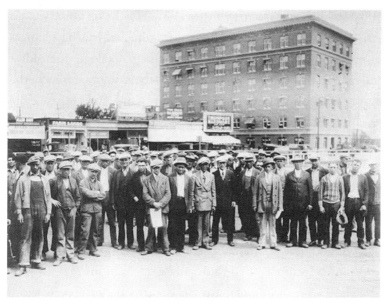

Group of local unemployed men during the Great Depression. LIBRARY AND
ARCHIVES CANADA C-020595.

to win a 48-hour work week for nurses. But in 1939 the first
strike in the history of BC nursing broke out in Comox, and
for one week nurses demonstrated for an eight-hour day and
two weeks of paid vacation every year.

For the Sisters of Providence the gloom was briefly lifted on
May 6, 1935, when in honour of the Silver Jubilee celebrations
of King George V and Queen Mary, Sister Justina, the superior
of Saint Mary's Hospital, was awarded the Golden Medal, and
it was presented to her at a large public ceremony at Queen's
Park. Then in June of the following year she was again honoured, this time by Mayor Hume and city council on the occasion of her transfer. Having helped so many of those affected
by the worst years of the Great Depression with every available

penny at the Sisters' disposal, she was presented with a small purse of money to encourage her at long last to keep a little bit of money for herself.

It was not until 1938 that economic conditions began to improve, and this was reflected in the fact that the hospital gave out only 1,096 meals to the poor that year. But the Depression had not ended the Sisters' commitment to keep up with modern hospital trends. Sister M. Patrick and Sister Maxima received formal training in administration in 1936, a large gas stove was installed in 1937, and a deep freeze was purchased in 1938. The next year saw the installation of a modern heating system, one that was automatic, where the temperature could actually be controlled by thermostats! And 1939 was prosperous enough for the hospital to receive a new coat of stucco— brown-red on the top floor and cream on the rest of the hospital and the nurses' home.

On April 12, 1940, Sister Charles Elisée and registered

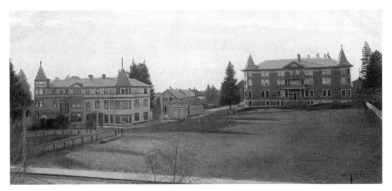

Columbian College. The Ladies' Building is to the left, the Men's Building to the right. Columbian College closed during the Great Depression but Saint Mary's made it through the period, thanks in large part to an arrangement that allowed for direct funding by the city. JAIMIE McEVOY PRIVATE COLLECTION.

nurse Therese Marie represented Saint Mary's at a meeting of the Catholic Hospital Association of British Columbia, which was affiliated with the larger North American organization. Although throughout the years Saint Mary's had been the institution that others had studied and the one that had received all the awards of excellence, this was the beginning of the Sisters' efforts to seek expertise and knowledge from other hospitals. With the modern era had come modern labour relations, and the Sisters of Providence, who saw their work as a Christian mission that at times required some personal sacrifice, found the nursing staff's new emphasis on wages and working conditions somehow out of place in Saint Mary's. But with the Depression at last over, nurses had begun to chafe under the restrictions of life attached to a hospital, unions were organizing and governments were adopting and enforcing new labour standards.

Up to this time the hospital had been charging room and board to the nurses who lived in the nurses' residence, but in April 1940 the Board of Labour pronounced the charge to be too high and ordered a refund for the past six months. At the same time the hospital was ordered not only to pay its maids the minimum wage but to back-pay it for the previous four months. Then in August the Wage Board ordered the hospital to pay graduate nurses a monthly salary of $75 plus room and board. The Sisters administering the hospital accepted this agreement, and then to further reduce tensions they eliminated the common dining room and provided separate apartments for nurses. They also installed separate restrooms for the nurses and the other employees of the hospital.

The following year the New Westminster Elks Club raised

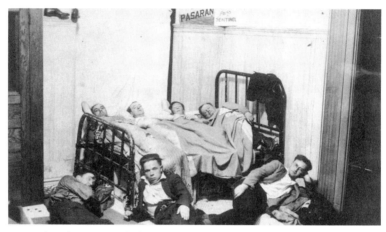

Unemployed men crowded into a shared rented room, circa 1930s. Crowded living conditions among the poor contributed to the prevalence of disease in neighbourhoods served by Saint Mary's Hospital. CBC, LIBRARY AND ARCHIVES CANADA C-013236.

funds for several items of hospital equipment and a new advisory board was formed. While the hospital had always been a partnership between the community and the Sisters of Providence, the new board now gave the community at large a say in governing the hospital. Mr. McClosky, a Grand Knight of Columbus, was the first chair.

Until this time World War II had seemed far away, but when on December 7, 1941, the Japanese bombed Pearl Harbor, it came frighteningly close to home. The next day, after Japanese planes were reported off the coast of Alaska, a full blackout was ordered in the City of New Westminster. Gallons of black paint, miles of black building paper, yards of black cloth and thousands of thumb tacks were acquired so that the hospital could be rendered invisible in its own black shroud. Fire-fighting carts were placed throughout the hallways to be

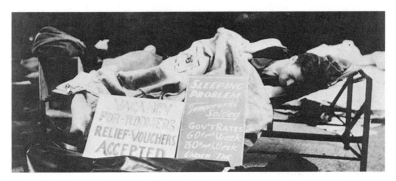

Man sleeping on cot during the Great Depression. LIBRARY AND ARCHIVES
CANADA C-020594.

ready in case bombs should fall. Gas masks were issued, and
at times Saint Mary's seemed like the ancient Christian cata-
combs as the Sisters knelt in the darkened hallways and in the
wards among the patients offering prayers for all to hear. For
the next two years a complete blackout was imposed and the
ban was not lifted until October 1943.

Rationing and shortages became the order of the day. By
order of the federal government the hospital's heating plant was
switched from oil to coal. For the nurses in the hospital, the
shortages had many practical effects. Although formal coffee
breaks had yet to be introduced—in fact, the eight-hour shift
was still a relatively recent improvement on the old twelve-
hour shifts, and nurses still only had one day off a week—it
was still possible from time to time to stop for a cup of coffee.
However, during the war that coffee had to be taken black,
without cream and sugar, and sometimes there was no coffee at
all. More importantly, great care had to be taken with medical
instruments because new parts were often unavailable, and doctors sometimes had to be creative when a necessary instrument

was broken. Perhaps most difficult was the shortage of medical staff as many doctors and nurses were serving overseas, and there were often tears at Saint Mary's as nurses mourned lost colleagues. But at the same time nursing schools were bursting with new students.

Just before Christmas 1938 Saint Mary's Hospital had been assigned a new superior. She was Sister Celina, who had been the superintendent of nurses at Saint Paul's School of Nursing, which provided many nurses for Saint Mary's. Even though anti-Japanese feeling was stirring in British Columbia as the result of the Japanese invasion of Manchuria and then China, in 1937 Sister Celina had ignored a decision of her governing board and put her own career at risk to admit two Japanese women as nursing students, and she made it clear that she hoped their time at the school would open a path for others to follow.

Thanks to the decision of Sister Celina, Dorothy Nakamachi and Norrie (Yamanaka) Ughetto would become registered nurses in 1940, in the same graduating class as Florence Hagarty, later to become known as the legendary Sister Mary Michael, who would serve as the superior of Saint Mary's Hospital through much of the 1960s and 1970s. Recalling her efforts to become a nurse, Dorothy Nakamachi wrote:

> In those early years, it was difficult for us to enter nursing in British Columbia. A United Church-affiliated hospital at Lamont in Alberta was the only place an Oriental girl could apply. Vancouver General Hospital had accepted the first Japanese-Canadians around 1934 but [they only took] one each year. In 1937 their quota was filled and Saint

Paul's had not opened its door to non-whites, so I applied to the hospital in Lamont. My parish priest was upset that a Catholic girl could not enter a Catholic hospital's school of nursing; he could not understand that there was also a racial bias involved. He went to the superintendent of nurses to appeal my case. As a result, the board of directors amended their policy and decided to accept one Oriental girl into the school. However, coincidentally just about that time, prior to my application, another had come from a Japanese-Canadian who was attending the University of British Columbia, [though she was] not a Catholic. Sister Celina [superintendent of nurses] told me later that they were faced with a problem because the one-entrant policy meant Norrie's (Noriko Yamanaka) application was the first and yet I, as a Catholic girl, also needed to be considered. So they decided to open the doors wide and accepted both of us!

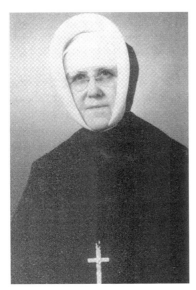

Sister Celina solemnly told us on the first day how much of a responsibility we had in setting a path for the future Asian girls that may be accepted on the basis of how

Sister Celina, superior at Saint Mary's Hospital from 1946 to 1951, who admitted the first nursing students of Japanese descent into Saint Paul's Hospital School of Nursing. PHOTOGRAPH COURTESY OF NEW WESTMINSTER MUSEUM AND ARCHIVES.

well we performed and the academic records we showed. It put an extra onus on Norrie and me, but after two years when they accepted another Japanese-Canadian girl, we felt that we had performed satisfactorily.

I think I can say for myself and perhaps for Norrie, too, that the basic nursing training and philosophy and ethic learned at Saint Paul's were the strong foundations on which we built our successful nursing careers. In spite of the many racial tensions I experienced due to the attitude of the society on the West Coast and a couple of unpleasant experiences I encountered while nursing, the Sisters of Charity of Providence were champions on our behalf and defended our rights.

Notable examples are shown by [what] our wonderful nursing director, Sister Columbkile [sic] did for the Japanese-Canadian nurses during the months immediately after Pearl Harbor. I was a graduate then and working on night shift. During those dark days the Japanese-Canadian community had curfews imposed on us, which made it difficult for me to go to work after sundown. Sister Columbkile gave me a room in the residence free of charge, which she said I could use from the time of sundown until I went on duty at 11 p.m. In this way I was able to continue working until the day I had to leave Vancouver because of the Evacuation Policy. Another thing Sister Columbkile did for the beleaguered JC [Japanese-Canadian] nurses was that she applied and received special permission from the BC Security Commission [the authority that administered the evacuation of the Japanese Canadians] to allow a JC student who was in her last year of training to stay until the deadline and during the six months before the final day of evacuation. Mitsu Shoyama was given all her theories and examinations and the final six months of practical training was arranged for her to be completed at a hospital in Alberta where she graduated as a Saint Paul's Hospital nurse.

If there had been a biased policy of racism in [the] early 1930s the Sisters of Providence certainly showed their compassion and understanding during [the] 1940s . . . I'm sure the hospital has opened its doors wider and wider during the 50-plus years to embrace all races and creeds and its expansion not only physically but in philosophy and medical skills has made it the great hospital it is today.

As measures against the Japanese increased after war broke out, a dusk-to-dawn curfew was declared for all persons of Japanese descent, even for doctors who were not even allowed to visit patients during the curfew. Muriel Kitagawa, who attended Connaught High School in New Westminster, writing about the events leading up to the expulsion of the Japanese, noted:

Witness the dying father and his daughter living in another part of the town who was prevented from going to his side, though she had pleaded to be allowed out, and the doctor who was unable to attend to that man because the curfew also kept him in . . . It was never our next-door neighbours that demanded expulsion for they knew us through daily contact. We felt a mutual respect and friendliness, and they were sincere in their sympathy for us.

When Japanese Canadians were subsequently interned, it was

a blow to Saint Mary's Hospital and its long relationship with that community. The Sisters, doctors and nurses at the hospital had known many of these people personally so they were vocal in their opposition to their removal from the coast, but thousands of them were interned and some 1,200 of their fishing boats were seized and sold at auction.

At the end of the war the old wooden Saint Mary's building got a major facelift. For those who worked at the hospital, the change was dramatic. "One can scarcely recognize Saint Mary's so great is the transformation," the *Chronicles* report.[47] Back in 1943 the landmark water tower had been removed as it had become loose and unsafe, and now the whole building got a fresh coat of paint, fancy new linoleum was installed and doors got a new coat of veneer. Cement steps replaced wooden ones, ceilings were lowered and the western stairwell was removed to expand the laboratory. In 1948 unused chimneys were removed to gain more space, a trend in old buildings throughout the city at that time. The nursery was enlarged and an X-ray unit was installed at a cost of about eleven thousand dollars, although over the years it was sometimes difficult to recruit an X-ray technician as they were so much in demand. Thanks to the Elks' continued fundraising, in 1949 a telephone switchboard was installed. (In earlier times when Saint Mary's had been one of the first buildings in New Westminster with a phone, the Sisters had raised a little money by charging locals who came to make telephone calls or to receive messages.)

Another branch of health care in New Westminster took a step forward in 1948 when the old Hollywood Sanitarium at the corner of Sixth Street and Fifth Avenue was sold to Dr. Ernest A. Campbell, who specialized in treating alcoholism and who began to include more of the common people and fewer of the elite. The next owner was Dr. J. Ross MacLean, who changed the name to Hollywood Hospital and again renovated the property. McLean continued to specialize in treating alcoholism but he also operated the hospital as a modern acute psychiatric clinic, treating all manner of mental illnesses. Patients were said to include ministers in the provincial government of W.A.C. Bennett, but many people referred to the institution were actually supported by Catholic charities.

The hospital became famous in a different way when Dr. MacLean began to experiment with psychedelic drugs as a method of treatment and published papers on the use of LSD and other drugs at the hospital. Some patients paid up to one thousand dollars per dose, although on average it would be five hundred to six hundred dollars, but MacLean claimed an 80 percent recovery rate from alcoholism with controlled treatments of LSD. Clientele soon included Canadian parliamentarians and American movie stars. Singer Andy Williams openly talked about having been a patient under LSD treatment there; said the crooner, "Maybe that's why I'm so cool."[48]

The Saint Mary's Hospital Society formed in 1915 had become dormant during the 1930s, but its intent was revived on February 11, 1947, when thirty-four women met to form the Saint Mary's Hospital Auxiliary. Membership cost one dollar. The purpose of the organization was simply "to find a way to add to the comfort and welfare of the patients of Saint Mary's Hospital,"[49] and on April 23 they began their efforts with a bazaar and tea, which raised $1,113. The Auxiliary quickly moved from its first contribution of a cozy rug for the Saint Mary's parlour to providing valuable medical services such as setting up the hospital's blood bank. They personally welcomed new patients and escorted them to their rooms, delivered books to the bedside and hosted teas on Wednesdays for palliative care patients and their families. They became known for the home-made afghans and quilts they provided for the beds and cots and family rooms where family members could be close to sick relatives. The women of the Auxiliary also ran the hospital gift shop and were generally involved in many other aspects of the hospital's activities.

A year after the Auxiliary's founding British Columbia's Liberal government under Byron Johnson introduced hospital insurance, and the first inspection of Saint Mary's under the new insurance scheme was made on August 3, 1949, by the Health Ministry's A.R. Simmons. He is reported to have left quite satisfied. The new schemes and the favourable inspection should have boded well for Saint Mary's as it promised to al-leviate financial pressures, but insurance benefits were limited to acute-care patients, and the hospital was still challenged by the large number of charitable patients admitted who needed chronic care. The Auxiliary then undertook to raise funds for services for which there was no government aid, and their main method was the "tag day." On most Saturdays, the members of the Auxiliary would be strategically stationed throughout the city asking the public to give a donation in exchange for a little paper tag. Wearing the tag meant that the person would not be approached to buy another tag that day. As always, these fund-raisers were a partnership between the hospital and the com-munity. The Royal Canadian Legion supplied the headquarters where the volunteers were co-ordinated and dispatched with military precision, and various community groups supported the effort by adopting a street corner. New volunteers were accompanied by more experienced canvassers to ensure that they learned the correct technique for "asking people to buy a tag and aid the cause."[50] The emphasis was placed on presentability and good manners. With costs averaging just twelve dollars for all the paper tags and the string to attach them to a coat button, the event usually brought in some five hundred to seven hundred dollars. As a result, this fundraising technique became too popular and city council found it necessary to step in and co-ordinate the dates.

The Auxiliary missed no opportunity to raise money, even deciding within their first year to charge ten cents per member for the refreshments served at their meetings, and a few months later when they were invited to attend the annual May Day celebrations, they decided to set up a booth to sell "ice cream sandwiches, orange crush, coca-cola, and doughnuts."[51] Bazaars that featured craft sales, raffles and home cooking brought the community into the hospital and provided patients with a welcome respite from illness. Prizes at the fish pond—just twenty-five cents a try—were the kittens of Bluey the cat, and to this day some still say that the hospital's official shade of blue was chosen because of Bluey.

Before the end of 1947 the energy and ambition of the Auxiliary members led to the establishment of the Marion Bakery at Kingsway and Tenth Avenue in the hope that the bakery profits would end the need for teas, bazaars, raffles and tag days. The women volunteers were organized into half-day shifts once a week, but while the bakery was successful it was only marginally so compared with the other fundraising efforts, and in the end it was sold.

The practical work of the Auxiliary was diverse and included everything from sewing and mending the hospital's sheets to conducting hospital tours. The women doubled their efforts at Christmastime by contributing jams and pickles, and some years they served turkey dinners at Dontenwill Hall, cooking the turkeys and apple pies at home and the potatoes in the hospital kitchen. A local cannery provided the vegetables. Every patient received a Christmas gift, and at Easter they decorated the pediatric ward, complete with Easter eggs from the Easter bunny.

During all of this, the women of the Auxiliary still found time to support the Local Council of Women and the Red Cross, canvass for donations for a forerunner to the United Way, contribute to the Vagabond Players theatrical group, raise money for the Cancer Fund and for emergencies such as the 1948 Fraser River Flood Relief Fund. They prepared for fu-

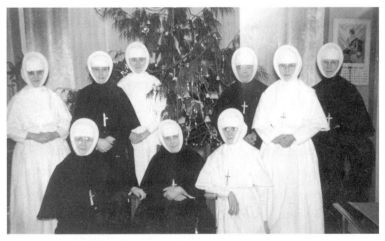

Sisters of Providence at Saint Mary's Hospital during a Christmas event. The nursing Sisters are wearing white, the other Sisters black. UNDATED PHOTOGRAPH COURTESY OF NEW WESTMINSTER MUSEUM AND ARCHIVES MANUSCRIPT #302.

ture emergencies by helping to organize mock disaster days. On two occasions they presented babies with the Auxiliary's rarest prize—a silver spoon; these went to the last baby born at the old hospital and the first born in the new hospital in 1958. There was also, of course, the important duty of welcoming the city's May Queen and entourage on her annual visit and hosting her tea.

The Auxiliary was not immune to outside events. When Mrs. L. McEvoy was elected the society's treasurer in 1950, she faced a particularly daunting task. Health-care costs were steadily rising, but funding from the government's hospital insurance plan was not adequate. Saint Mary's was receiving $10 per day per patient from the provincial government; the patient paid an extra $1.75 to $4, but, when the patient couldn't pay, this amount had to be absorbed by the hospital. (The Vancouver General was receiving $13.50 per day per patient from the government at this time.) While this insurance was certainly an improvement on the government's previous unreliable grant program, public debate on the subject became so heated that the Auxiliary decided to suspend its tag days and other public fundraising events because, whenever its members were out canvassing on street corners, they were drawn into arguments about health-care funding. Without the tag days, however, the Auxiliary could not meet its fundraising goals. Mrs. McEvoy's solution was to double the members' cost for meeting refreshments to twenty cents—and the goals were met.

Meanwhile, the hospital's modernization process had continued into the 1950s. More Sisters were formally trained in administration, and in 1953 Sister Adelard Clement, who had been trained as a dietitian, arrived to take over the hospital kitchens. The Sisters, whose order had always understood and emphasized the importance of good nourishment, welcomed this new addition to their staff as she would ensure that meals were prepared to the highest standards possible. In addition to the work of the Sisters and nurses themselves, in the 1950s the hospital also began to hire more women for other important positions; in 1953 Elizabeth Epping was hired as X-ray technician and Mrs. R. Barrows as laboratory technician.

On December 14, 1952, the Sisters celebrated the completion of the new chapel with its aquamarine walls and ceiling, the colour that would become so closely identified with Saint Mary's. The new organ was installed in time to be played by Sister Patricia Ann on Christmas Eve.

7

The New Saint Mary's Hospital

ALL THE IMPROVEMENTS TO SAINT MARY'S HOSPITAL during the 1940s and 1950s had made it more efficient, but each improvement had also further overtaxed the crowded little building, even though the original 1887 wooden structure had been expanded many times. There had been an addition in 1912, more space had been gained when the nurses' living quarters had been freed up after their new accommodations were built in 1928, the wards had been redesigned to add more beds, and chimneys and stairwells had been removed to expand labs, but by the 1950s none of this was enough. What was needed was a completely modern new building to replace the sixty-five-year-old one, and on May 7, 1953, the Mother House of the Sisters of Providence in Montreal gave approval for an investigation into the possibility of constructing it.

The old hospital had served the community well. From its opening day on May 25, 1887, to December 31, 1957, the little hospital that started with forty-two beds had admitted 72,601 patients. It had housed an unknown number of homeless, given temporary shelter to hundreds of disaster victims, fed the hungry, and saved the lives of many who would otherwise have succumbed. A conservative estimate is that at least eighty thousand meals had been served to the poor by a staff that rarely exceeded ten people. At no point had the reputation or the work of the hospital ever faltered because the Sisters and the community had faced every challenge together. It made sense, then, when it came time to replace the old Saint Mary's, to build it on these same twin pillars—the Sisters of Providence and the community—formalizing a partnership that had for so long been so successful.

New Westminster's Mayor Toby Jackson, who also served as chair of the hospital board, wrote the necessary letters and made contact with the BC Health Insurance Services (BCHIS) to promote the new building, and by October 1953 Donald Cox and E.W.J. Pitkethley from BCHIS had inspected the grounds and agreed that the old orchard beside the present building would provide a suitable site for a new hospital. On June 10, 1954, Jackson and four other members of the board met with Premier W.A.C. Bennett to request that the province put up 50 percent of the costs of construction. Bennett was reassuring and offered "a promising message to Sister Leo Francis, Superior." But the following spring when Sister Leo Francis and Sister Margaret of Charity met with BCHIS Commissioner Donald Cox, they found that, although he was willing to support a new hospital, he was not willing to grant 175 beds, the number Saint Mary's representatives had identified as necessary, based on a health-care needs survey of the area.

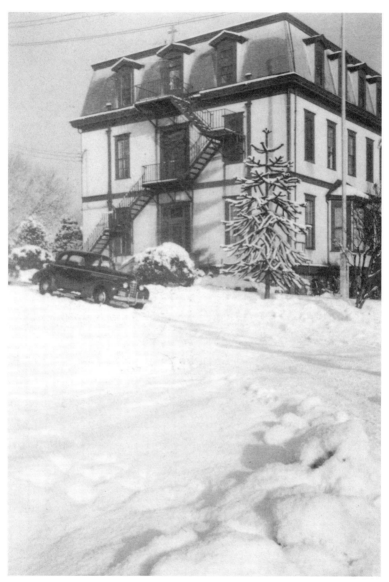

An elevator, fire escape, electric lights and a fashionable monkey puzzle
tree all show change from the hospital's construction in 1887. But Saint
Mary's needed to build a completely new hospital to greet the modern
era. PHOTOGRAPH COURTESY OF NEW WESTMINSTER MUSEUM AND ARCHIVES IHP7852.

And thus was instituted a pattern that would last for the next fifty years—Saint Mary's Hospital would stubbornly insist on receiving support based on the medical needs of the community and government officials would emphasize cost as their primary consideration.

On February 16, 1955, funding was finally approved for 150 beds instead of the necessary 175. Then on March 5, despite an understanding achieved only a few weeks earlier, Victoria returned the plans with significant alterations: the kitchen, cafeteria, laboratory and surgical preparation areas had all been reduced in size below the architects' and medical professionals' recommendations. Worse, the government had agreed to allow an emergency department to be built but, very oddly, would not fund it once it was in place. This would leave the hospital with an empty and unused emergency department in a brand new building.

The hospital board and Sister Leo Francis reacted to the changed plans by uniting in their resistance; they decided that they simply would not conform to Victoria's decision. Fortunately, although officials in the Ministry of Health never did agree to back down, in the end they were forced to approve construction in accordance with the design approved by Saint Mary's board because they were instructed to do so by Minister of Health Eric Martin, who had been subjected to considerable political pressure. However, while the hospital had won the battle, within the ranks of Victoria's bureaucracy, Saint Mary's staff and board were now regarded as troublemakers.

On November 10 the hospital and the city of New Westminster were swept by excitement when a telegram arrived giving final government approval for construction. Taking no chances that the ministry would change its collective mind again, the board let out tenders almost immediately, and Bennett and White were quickly selected as the contractors. On December 15, Judge H. Sullivan, the new board chair, ceremonially turned the first sod on what had been the old orchard behind the hospital. Fundraising by the Elks, the Women's Auxiliary and others went into high gear. In August 1956 Robinson Construction was awarded the general contract for $1,698,000, with Barr and Anderson receiving a second contract of $553,403 for plumbing, heating and ventilation.

Many in the community thought the hospital would now be built as planned, but it was never that easy for Saint Mary's. By March 1957 it became clear that the Mother House could no longer provide loans and, as a result, financing the portion of costs beyond the province's contribution became a real challenge for the new superior sister, Rose Wilfreda, and the board. However, even with only half-funding by the province and no money available from the Mother House, they awarded contracts in April in the amount of $326,346 to Mott Electrical Ltd. In June there were more challenges when the hospital's employees unionized "much to the regret of the Sisters."[52] The challenges were becoming more and more immense and costs would continue to increase. But good news also came that month when Sister Anne Alberta, the provincial treasurer of the Sisters of Providence, announced that the order had been able to secure a loan from the Royal Bank of Canada to complete the construction. This happy news was balanced on July 3, 1957, by a letter from the BCHIS informing the hospital's administration that a per diem patient rate had been approved at $13.25 per day, rather than the requested $14. This meant that Saint Mary's would operate at a deficit just to provide basic services to patients. It was, however, not at all uncommon at that time—when most BC hospitals still had community boards and operated independently—for their administrators to make decisions based on health-care needs and, as a result, incur deficits. Ultimately, effective cost-cutting as a priority would be part of the reason the government began to phase out hospital boards, place hospitals under the control of regional health authorities and bring in business people as administrators. But in 1957 Saint Mary's was operating much as any other hospital when it came to funding, which was to do what was in the best interest of patients.

Construction of the new Saint Mary's continued through the fall of 1957. When the day came for the life-sized statue of Saint Mary to be removed from the entrance to the old hospital and installed on the new one, the New Westminster Fire Department, with its long relationship with Saint Mary's, was entrusted with the job. Four firefighters scaled the ladder from the fire truck to do it, and this was viewed by the Sisters as "an unusual act of gallantry."[53] Then as the final coat of aquamarine paint was applied, Sister Leo Francis announced that she was extraordinarily proud of her "blue baby." Saint Mary's patients were moved into the new building on November 1, 1957. Not since the Great Fire of 1898 or the blackouts of World War II had there been such a challenging day, because the patients' needs didn't suddenly stop for the event. The last baby born in the old hospital was a girl to Mrs. A. Wilkies at 2:23 a.m. Mrs. J. Fielder's baby boy was the first born in the new hospital at 4:48 p.m. Both babies were delivered by Dr. G.I. Piercy. It would be November 4 before things would settle down enough for Father Stephen Murphy, OMI, to perform mass in the temporary chapel in the new auditorium, but this was probably the most suitable place, after all, since Saint Mary's had always been as much a gathering place for the community as it was a hospital.

In January 1959 the manner in which the hospital was administered changed forever. The Sisters remained the owners, but the decision-making authority for it was transferred to the board. This was an entirely suitable move since the hospital had managed for more than seventy years on funds raised largely by the local, mostly non-Catholic community and with the political leadership and support of local citizens. Community representatives such as Mayor Toby Jackson, Justice Sullivan and others now worked to formalize this partnership, and hospital board vice-chairman and lawyer G. McKinnon worked with Sister Denise Marguerite to

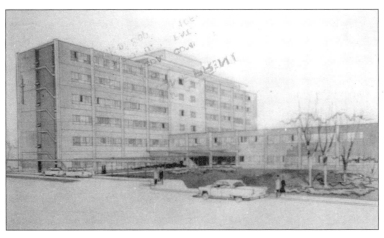

An artist's rendering of the new Saint Mary's Hospital circa 1957. IMAGE COURTESY OF NEW WESTMINSTER MUSEUM AND ARCHIVES MANUSCRIPT #302.

formulate a new constitution and bylaws. The City of New Westminster appointed its newly elected "lady Mayor" Beth Wood to the hospital board and the Sisters appointed former Mayor Toby Jackson as their representative. In March Judge Sullivan resigned as board chair and Jackson took his place. In short order this new governing structure for the hospital was approved by the Minister of Health.

However, although Saint Mary's, while still owned by a Catholic order, was now operated by a community board and integrated into the regional and provincial health-care system, it would never be treated routinely as if it were part of the provincial system. It was always regarded by the province's bureaucracy as an anomaly, even though most governments in other jurisdictions, no matter their political stripe, generally appreciate religious hospitals because of their land base, experience and generally frugal not-for-profit nature. In fact, in the years to come, the integration that Saint Mary's continued to seek, while still maintaining a degree of independence, would become the norm in the rest of North America, and today almost half of all North American hospital patients are still treated at Catholic charity institutions. But while at times Saint Mary's relationship with health officials in British Columbia would improve, at other times it would not, with the result that Saint Mary's full acceptance into the public health-care system never took place and it would rarely be encouraged or given the opportunity to grow. This did not stop Saint Mary's from continuing to change and innovate—largely by creating such opportunities for itself and often by exercising its political support to achieve its goals—and it continued to annoy health bureaucrats who didn't think much of small hospitals, Catholic

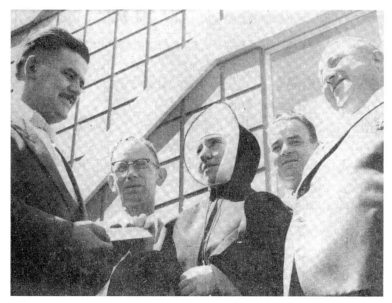

Money was raised by many community groups for Saint Mary's Hospital.
THE BRITISH COLUMBIAN, JULY 14, 1958, COURTESY OF NEW WESTMINSTER PUBLIC LIBRARY.

hospitals, those run by women and/or community boards or those that fitted into other newly proscribed categories.

On June 26, 1959, the interior of the chapel was finally finished. It was three years, seven months and three days since Justice Sullivan had turned the first sod. However, even though the hospital was now officially fully complete, the province of British Columbia had still not paid its portion of the construction costs. Its final payment for construction did not arrive until 1965, fully nine years after the first contracts had been awarded.

While in the early days Saint Mary's had served primarily as a hospital for injured working men and at times as a disaster-relief hospital, after 1905 when Women's Hospital had been absorbed by the Royal Columbian, maternity had very gradually become increasingly important at Saint Mary's, and after 1959 babies and children would be a very large part of the hospital's mission. Thus it was very appropriate that in August 1959 Minister of Health Eric Martin approved alterations to expand the department of pediatrics, and the entire third floor with its fifty-three beds was now dedicated to the care of children. At the same time the hospital's total bed capacity was increased from 150 to 171. The Women's Auxiliary played a critical role at this point, raising money for nursery equipment, humidifiers, infant resuscitators, oxygen tents, incubators for premature babies, defibrillators, physiotherapy equipment and a new blood bank. They also provided a lawn mower and ice cubes. By 1968, the Auxiliary was contributing $11,000 annually, and by 1986 it had raised a total of $250,000 for the hospital. However, even as the Auxiliary was proving to be a powerhouse of fundraising, the 1960s also saw a growing number

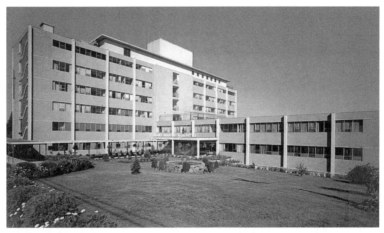

Postcard of the newly constructed Saint Mary's Hospital. IMAGE COURTESY OF NEW WESTMINSTER MUSEUM AND ARCHIVES.

of bequests from former patients. In addition, the regional role of Saint Mary's led to grants from the municipality of Coquitlam, and donations also came in from groups like the New Westminster Medical Association.

On the staffing front, the 1960s introduced superannuation; after July 1, 1960, female employees would be retired at the age of sixty, male employees at the age of sixty-five. Women employees often remarked that this arrangement was more than fair on the grounds that they did most of the work anyway.

After the hospital's first eye surgery took place on November 16, 1960, performed by Dr. E.F. Amhalt on patient Montague Grant, Saint Mary's increasingly became known for its ophthalmology. Rehabilitative physiotherapy also became a specialty and contributed to Saint Mary's Hospital becoming a preferred location for orthopaedic surgery. A medical library was established and catalogued by Sister Denise Marguerite.

In 1962 formal accreditation began under the Canadian Council of Accreditation, and the hospital received full accreditation on August 22. However, just one year later, Saint Mary's had again run out of space, and the board began to look for support for an expansion that would provide more beds. On March 26 the chief of staff, L.S. Chipperfield, made a public call for one hundred more medical and surgical beds, and the expansion plans were approved in principle by the board on May 28, just two months later. Fortunately, the hospital continued to have strong support at this time in political circles, as demonstrated by the donation from the will of a former Lieutenant-Governor of BC, Randolph Bruce, in the amount of $12,935.75, and the Mother House, which made the final decisions on all matters involving construction, then granted permission to use this bequest as the start of a new building fund. There was understandable disappointment, therefore, when in April 1964 the Mother House informed the hospital's superior, Mary Michael, who had taken over as head on November 15, 1962, that no funds were available to assist with the construction project. Fortunately, during this period, relations with health officials were mostly positive because Saint Mary's was showing excellent results, it was popular with patients, and it was one of the newest hospital facilities in the entire region—all facts that were appreciated by health authorities in the 1960s. As a result, the Hospital Area Planning Group, having investigated the location and the demographics, agreed to give Saint Mary's top priority for expansion to meet the acute bed shortage, and former mayor F.H. Jackson was named to look at ways to raise funds for all of the hospitals seeking new construction in the region. In this way competition for resources was set aside in favour of working with the abilities of the other hospitals, which benefited from Saint Mary's political and community support. This was the high point in regional co-operation and benefited the health-care system and all the hospitals over a large area.

Meanwhile, Saint Mary's continued to improve its services to its patients. The death from cancer of the well-liked hospital superior, Sister Rose Wilfreda, in 1963 at Saint Paul's Hospital, encouraged a strong interest in tackling that disease with the latest techniques and equipment. By July the hospital had taken steps to purchase a freezing microtome machine, allowing for the early detection of cancer cells in biopsies. For the rest of its life, Saint Mary's placed a high priority on keeping up to date in the field of cancer detection and early treatment.

About this time Sister Superior Mary Michael, who was an accomplished administrator, was elected to the position of second vice-president of the BC Hospitals Association, the first Catholic Sister ever to sit on the organization's executive committee. Then on August 22, 1964, Health Minister Eric Martin finally gave approval to the board to construct a new wing that would accommodate eighty-four more beds, and the Sisters of Providence gave approval for the raising of additional funds through a city bylaw. A lot was purchased at 200 Royal Avenue, and land for parking was purchased at a cost of $18,000. A.C. Smith, who had been the architect of the new hospital and of New Westminster's City Hall eight years earlier, was hired to design the addition, and a twenty-page action plan was prepared after consultation, not only with administration, but also with Saint Mary's doctors and nurses. The City of New Westminster was involved in a practical way from the outset, paying the architect's bill of $20,000.

Saint Mary's *Chronicles* for 1964 state, "In terminating the chronicle of the events for the past year, the annalist records that, although the hospital continues to operate through deficit financing on the material plane, it enjoys, nevertheless, a rich and inexhaustible treasury of spiritual reserves. Because of the devoted efforts of the Sister Supervisors and Oblate Priests, the patients continually express their gratitude for the countless acts of charity and spiritual assistance rendered on their behalf during the period of their hospitalization. The comforting thought makes all else worthwhile."[54]

A sad day for Saint Mary's came on February 17, 1966, when Frederick John Hume, the Depression-era mayor of New Westminster, died at the age of 75. Hume's efforts had helped

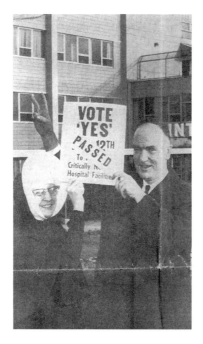

Hospital Administrator Sister Superior Mary Michael and Mayor Stuart Gifford celebrate the passing of the hospital expansion bylaw, allowing the construction of a new hospital wing at Saint Mary's to move ahead. *THE BRITISH COLUMBIAN*, AUGUST, 1964, COURTESY OF NEW WESTMINSTER MUSEUM AND ARCHIVES.

the Royal City through those bad years and ensured that Saint Mary's would survive that difficult time to serve future generations. But the world was changing and, as it did, so did the Catholic Church and the Sisters of Providence. The weather-worn statue of Our Lady of the Immaculate Conception that had stood for sixty years outside the hospital—a statue that legend says had been carved by the renowned Mother Joseph herself—was replaced. Edmonton, Alberta, became the new headquarters of the Sisters of Providence in Western Canada with the construction there of Providence Centre. And, on September 23, 1966, the Sisters left behind the traditional nun's habit and began wearing street clothes and a simple head covering. So many people asked to see the new look or shyly took a peek at the Sisters that by 10:00 a.m. they decided to assemble and tour the hospital as a group, patiently visiting every part of the hospital and answering questions. However, it took two full hours to satisfy everyone, so ingrained was the sight of the old nun's habit. Most of their viewers favoured the change, although some regretted the loss of the familiar tradition. Among the Sisters, the new look was not universally welcomed but it was accepted as part of the changing times.

Construction on the new addition began on May 25, 1966, under the supervision of engineer John E. Pierce. (Sadly, Pierce died shortly after the project was completed, reviving memories of the death of Thomas McKay, the architect and builder of the first hospital back in 1887.) The *Chronicles* reported that "Both patients and staff are subsequently fascinated witnessing the activities of the sure-footed steelworkers as they scamper along

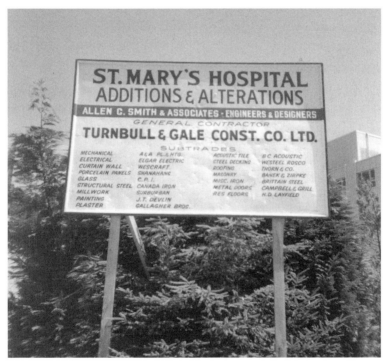

Allen C. Smith designed Saint Mary's Hospital and New Westminster City Hall. PHOTOGRAPH COURTESY OF NEW WESTMINSTER MUSEUM AND ARCHIVES.

the steel girders without any hesitation or fear."[55] A new front entrance to the hospital was opened by December 22, just in time for Christmas, and as usual the Sisters and nurses visited all the patients with gifts supplied by the Auxiliary. But the best Christmas present didn't arrive until January 1967 when the federal government approved grants of $263,733.34 toward construction costs, and work on the addition continued with a ten-ton boiler hoisted into place in late February.

The official opening of the hospital's addition occurred on October 28, 1967, and the *Chronicles* note the day with simple satisfaction: "The day is beautiful, the ceremony impressive and the crowds great."[56] The first patient in the newly opened addition was Mrs. Dorothy Orchard who was admitted by Dr. I.A. Bowie on November 1. Eighty-five new staff had been hired, and payment had been made in full to contractors by June 6, 1968, but note was taken in the *Chronicles* that, "the federal and provincial governments have yet to pay their final share of the construction costs."[57] In fact, the federal portion was not received until April 1969, and the provincial government didn't issue a cheque until August of that year. But the good news was that BCHIS funding had been increased to a per diem rate of $29.75 per patient.

Saint Mary's was now prepared for an uneventful few decades. But this was not to be. There were some routine matters, of course. New accreditation standards established in 1970 meant that the six-member medical executive committee would be replaced by a larger medical advisory committee representing heads of different departments and that the positions of chief of staff and president of the medical staff would be separated. A department of general practice was set up, and although it had largely been the case for many years, doctors were now made formally responsible for the quality of patient care in the hospital. More parcels of property were purchased for future expansion, including the old Kenny home across from the hospital on Hospital Street, 122 Royal Avenue, the Gehrer property and the Moore property. However, until the day when more expansion would occur, most of this newly acquired land was used to address the never-ending problem of where to park cars.

Money continued to come from the Elks for items such as a pressure preset ventilator for those suffering from acute respiratory problems and for pulmonary function equipment. The Royal Canadian Legion also made substantial donations

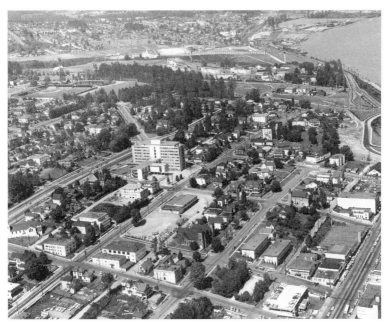

The new Saint Mary's Hospital dominated the city's skyline. PHOTOGRAPH COURTESY OF NEW WESTMINSTER MUSEUM AND ARCHIVES.

over the years, and every February the Auxiliary presented the hospital with a cheque for $10,000 and some years as much as $15,000. Despite the initial upset when employees had unionized, for the most part Saint Mary's Hospital had good employee relations in the 1960s, and the Sisters accepted with equanimity the 17.3 percent increase in wages won by the Hospital Employees' Union Local 180 in 1967. Saint Mary's was obviously a good place to work, and the *Chronicles* made note of several employees who had given twenty-five years or more of continual service. For Sister Paul, the inauguration of automated paycheques in 1969 was a tremendous boon since the staff now numbered four hundred and she could issue all four hundred paycheques in just fifteen minutes.

However, the 1970s were not routine. On April 6, 1970, the Minister of Health and Hospital Insurance, Ralph Loffmark, circulated a letter instructing all hospitals in British Columbia to reduce costs in order to finance a 30-percent increase in hospital salaries. The government had approved the increase but had decided not to fund it and was now expecting hospitals to come up with the necessary funds. The *Chronicles* report that "Saint Mary's Hospital administration, on the advice of its board of directors, decided to continue implementing its traditional philosophy of providing quality care through carefully controlled costs at all levels of operations."[58] Shortly after this, Loffmark toured the hospital and urged the hospital board and management to continue surgical day-care and to continue to buy land for expansion. Then he specifically encouraged them to look to intermediate and extended care. His comments about surgery and expansion were seen quite positively; few at that time gave much thought to his comments about extended care for the elderly.

Before the year was out, controversy once again surrounded the hospital and the role of the Catholic health-care system. On October 8, 1970, the *Columbian* newspaper ran a front-page article on the hospital's very public opposition to therapeutic abortions, a stand that threw the hospital once again into direct confrontation with the provincial government. In a televised address, the Minister of Health, who had just recently hinted that Saint Mary's should look to extended care, stated that hospitals supported by public funds "will have to face up to their public responsibilities in the area of abortions."[59] In return, the hospital's superior, Sister Mary Michael, emphasized that, while Saint Mary's had a community board, it was not a hospital society but a privately owned institution under an act of law—the Sisters of Providence in British Columbia Act of 1892. She argued that this Act had given the hospital the right to act according to its own philosophy. According to the *Chronicles*, the *Columbian* did not defend the hospital's views on abortion, but it did defend the hospital. "The editor, although a pro-abortion advocate, defended at some length the right of the corporately owned Catholic hospitals to operate according to their own moral philosophy. This is the first time that the local paper has ever defended the rights of Saint Mary's Hospital."[60]

The issue was of critical importance, not only in regards to the issue of abortion. Saint Mary's hoped to steadfastly refuse to perform therapeutic abortion services while still continuing to receive public and community support for the medical services that it was providing. The newspaper and others who wanted expanded access to abortions suggested that it was unnecessary to require Catholic hospitals to allow abortions because there were enough other hospitals willing to do so and because, although no one said so publicly, there was some real doubt whether Catholic hospitals would be willing to continue to exist if forced to perform abortions. If Catholic hospitals decided to close rather than comply, it would have caused a real crisis in the provision of health care. So the debate raged on, while Catholic hospitals continued to refuse to comply with the minister's demands. Once again, Saint Mary's increased its reputation for non-conformity.

A year later there was a new move to make Saint Mary's give up its independence when the Royal Columbian Hospital initiated talks on amalgamation. The overture was firmly rejected by the Saint Mary's Hospital board, and "relief was expressed by the majority of doctors."[61] The hospital continued to operate as a Catholic hospital, broadcasting morning and evening prayers over its public-address system, and the Sisters continued to visit patients to give encouragement and spiritual support. It was noted that many non-religious patients told the Sisters that they found the spiritual activities of the hospital comforting.

Meanwhile, though Saint Mary's was once again considered a troublemaker, it was maintaining its excellent reputation. In 1972 the BC Institute of Technology (BCIT) selected it as a teaching hospital for the Institute's first- and second-year nursing students, and the hospital's rehabilitative physiotherapy department, which was accredited by the Canadian Physiotherapy Association, was designated a teaching centre. In 1973 the hospital initiated a diabetic day-care program, approved by NDP Health Minister Dennis Cocke.

However, there were minuses, too. Although a merger with Royal Columbian had been rejected, that hospital began to absorb many of Saint Mary's medical programs. It began early in 1975 when the Ministry of Health transferred all emergency services to the Royal Columbian, and Saint Mary's emergency department became an out-patient service. But it was the loss of obstetrics to the Royal Columbian that was the hardest blow for Saint Mary's because it ended a seventy-year history as a place where babies were born. As early as 1974 Saint Mary's had been pressured to close its maternity ward in preparation for expansion at the Royal Columbian, but the hospital's obstetrical unit refused to wind down until the other hospital was actually ready to meet the demand. By October 1975, however, the medical advisory committee at Saint Mary's agreed to the transfer with the hospital board's decision to phase out the maternity ward as part of regional planning. Although many conflicting reasons were given to the public for the relocation of Saint Mary's obstetric services, in reality the hospital had seen declining admissions for childbirth for many years; in 1973 alone there had been a 21-percent decrease in newborn babies over the previous year, and accordingly beds had been reduced from 256 to 252 to compensate. At the same time there had been an increasing demand for surgery. In fact, at one point government logic had actually declared an overabundance of admissions for surgery, so the four-room labour unit was converted into the hospital's surgical day-care centre. It was largely accepted at Saint Mary's that the relatively low admissions in previous years were justification for this change as part of regional health strategy, and the hospital hoped to gain new support since it was now fully integrated into the regional public health-care system. In 1977 the hospital expanded its mandate to provide compassionate care by opening a social-service department.

8

Surviving the Provincial Government
1980–1996

"Up until now, we've been playing a gentleman's game. But we're beginning to doubt the gentlemen involved."

—GORDON BRUNSKILL,

CHAIR OF SAINT MARY'S HOSPITAL BOARD, 1980

SAINT MARY'S HOSPITAL WAS ACCUSTOMED to assaults on its right to exist as an acute-care hospital, but as its centennial approached, it faced its most serious threat since the lean days of 1910. But this was a strange time for this crisis to arise. Compared with most hospitals in Greater Vancouver, Saint Mary's was considered fairly new—a new building had replaced the original wooden structure in 1959 and a new wing was added in 1967—and under the firm hand of Sister Mary Michael, it was cost-effective and efficient. So the announcement by British Columbia's new Health Minister Rafe Mair that Saint Mary's would be changed from a fully operational acute-care hospital to an extended-care facility came as a shock to the hospital's staff and patients.

Mair's rationale for the change was that there were enough acute-care beds in the region but not enough extended-care facilities. His plan was to move Saint Mary's aside to make way for the recently approved $37-million Eagle Ridge Hospital project in Port Moody. Mayor Muni Evers and the New Westminster City Council publicly opposed the government's plans and called on the community to fight to keep Saint Mary's status as it was. The mayor argued the hospital's case to the media, always emphasizing that wait-lists at Saint Mary's were often only three weeks for elective surgery, and he stressed the fact that the hospital's modern role as an integrated part of the health-care system serving a large part of the Lower Mainland worked in support of the services offered by the Royal Columbian Hospital.

Evers was also highly critical of the Greater Vancouver Regional District (GVRD) Board who had made the decision in camera to approve the Eagle Ridge hospital project. "I strongly object to dispensing some $40 million of the taxpayers' money behind closed doors,"[62] he said. According to the mayor, the option that had been placed on the GVRD table to build Eagle Ridge and to phase out Saint Mary's was one and the same, and while he didn't object to a new hospital, he did not support phasing out Saint Mary's in the process. He said that it made no sense to build a hospital in one place and close a perfectly good existing hospital nearby while spending $40 million to accomplish the task.

Community groups in New Westminster, including the Twelfth Street Businessmen's Association led by Calvin

Donnelly, moved quickly to back Evers and Saint Mary's Hospital. Soon several groups in the city were writing letters to the Health Minister. "It's the only thing the provincial ministers listen to so we gave them something to chew on," said Donnelly.[63] And Saint Mary's Hospital became a hot topic in the provincial legislature. When New Westminster's NDP Member of the Legislature, Dennis Cocke, who described the proposed changes to Saint Mary's as "stupid,"[64] grilled Health Minister Mair on the planned changes, Mair denied he had asked that the previous Friday's meeting of the GVRD be held in secret. Cocke insisted that the minister's own task force on health care opposed the recommendation to convert Saint Mary's from a hospital to an extended-care facility, but when Mair was asked to table the task force's report in the legislature, he deferred, stating that much of the report was "sensitive."[65] (More than twenty-five years later when Mair was interviewed for this book, he remarked that Cocke "was Opposition critic and wouldn't be expected to do anything else. He was full of bull.")[66]

From the beginning of this battle, the hospital had the advantage in the local media but there were problems. The media consistently ignored the fact that the existing hospital was only twenty-three years old and often referred to it as a ninety-four-year-old institution. To the uninformed, this gave the impression that the hospital itself was out of date. In a media conference in July, Saint Mary's chief of staff, Dr. Irwin Stewart, announced that all the doctors on the hospital's medical advisory committee and the surgical and medical departments would oppose the conversion of the hospital. He also told the media that Saint Mary's maintained a better average wait time for surgery than any of the area's other hospitals because it did not have an emergency department that impacted the elective surgical caseload. Doctors, Stewart explained, are not in competition between hospitals and the doctors of Saint Mary's did not see themselves as in competition with Eagle Ridge or Royal Columbian Hospital. But he pointed out that in 1979 some two hundred doctors at Saint Mary's had seen eleven thousand patients from all over the province. Saint Mary's had highly developed specialties in ophthalmology, ear, nose and throat, urology and plastic surgery, and he cautioned that these specialties could not just be picked up and easily moved somewhere else. Then Stewart embarrassed the government by revealing that in April the Deputy Minister of Health, in a meeting with the hospital's medical heads, had warned that the construction of Eagle Ridge would result in the conversion of Saint Mary's to an extended-care facility. (And twenty-four years later he explained to this writer that "the doctors were told at the time to keep this quiet.")

The provincial government may have thought they could incur the wrath of Saint Mary's advocates and get away with it, even with formidable critics such as Mayor Evers and the medical establishment, but they had not anticipated Sister Mary Michael, who had been the administrator of Saint Mary's Hospital since the day the new hospital opened. A competent and tough administrator, she is fondly remembered for her tireless energy and commitment to patients and staff. "She used to count the pencils every morning," a former Saint Mary's employee jokingly recalled, and another said, "She was the last to bed at night and the first up every morning."

Even Rafe Mair was impressed. "One of the toughest birds I've ever met in my life," he recalled. "She was really tough and was the organization behind the whole fight. I took a liking to her because she was so spunky." In fact, he had really underestimated the religious opposition to the downgrading of Saint Mary's, saying that he hadn't realized that would be part of the opposition until he got into it. "I received enormous abuse. I couldn't go near a hospital without picket signs, and priests were railing at the pulpit."[67] Mair finally went to talk to Archbishop James Carney, arguing that the conversion of Saint Mary's was not a Catholic–Protestant issue, and he asked the Archbishop to "lay off."[68]

Meanwhile, Bill Vander Zalm, a Catholic who served in the same Social Credit Cabinet as Mair, began actively lobbying the government to change its position on Saint Mary's Hospital. The opposition to the government's decision now included the Roman Catholic Church, the City of New Westminster, the medical community, the strong NDP Opposition including the local MLA Dennis Cocke, most of the public, and now some members of the government caucus. Health Minister Mair's initial reaction was to push ahead, and he wrote to Saint Mary's board to advise them that they should prepare to convert the hospital to an extended-care facility over the next four years— the time it would take to build Eagle Ridge Hospital.

"Up until now, we've been playing a gentleman's game," said Gordon Brunskill, chair of the hospital board, "but we're beginning to doubt the gentlemen involved."[69] And the doctors continued to add fuel to the fire. Dr. Stewart publicly proclaimed that the loss of Saint Mary's as a hospital would cause "waiting lists like you've never seen in your life."[70]

When Mair fired back that the priorities in provincial health care were changing from acute care to extended care,

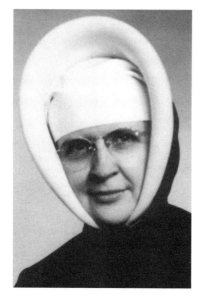

Sister Mary Michael led the fight against Rafe Mair and fought to keep Saint Mary's as an acute-care hospital. *THE COLUMBIAN*, JULY 11, 1980, B3.

Sister Mary Michael told him, "We have a distinguished record as an active acute-care hospital and that's the role we'd like to keep and it's the role the public would like to see us keep."

Pressure on Mair increased when the local members of his Social Credit Party went on the attack and warned that the government would be punished at the polls if he persisted in his plans for Saint Mary's. Alderman Mal Hughes, who had run unsuccessfully as a Social Credit candidate in New Westminster in the previous provincial election, told him that the conversion of Saint Mary's Hospital would "make Social Crediters an endangered species in this city . . . It's the worst political decision to affect New Westminster in a long time."[71] Hughes then moved a motion that was passed by city council demanding that Mair meet with council and the hospital board. In mid-August, Mayor Evers approached Mair at the official launch of a $42-million construction project to add 110 new acute-care beds to the Royal Columbian Hospital and wryly commented that this opening did not seem in keeping with the government's insistence that health care in the area was moving away from acute care to long-term care.

A petition that circulated in New Westminster collected 20,000 signatures in favour of keeping Saint Mary's as an acute-care facility, but Alderman Ken Wright noted that many of the signatures came from Burnaby and Surrey, indicating that there was just as much support for Saint Mary's Hospital in those areas as there was in New Westminster. The positive results of petitions circulated in other areas also contradicted the government's attempt to portray the matter as just a local New Westminster issue. However, Mair was unmoved by the petitions and responded to each petitioner with a letter stating only that the decision was made in the best interests of patients. In an interview in 2005 he commented that "there were more people signing petitions than there were living in BC. I felt the decision was right, but oh, there were scads of petitions . . . I give full marks to those who signed them saying they didn't want something and participating in the democratic process . . . New West was solid NDP so we weren't going to lose anything there anyway."[72]

But while Mair was unmoved, other politicians were not. Unlike today, local elected politicians had a strong say in health care and the process of health planning in their areas, and on September 24 hospital board chair Gordon Brunskill gave an eloquent and passionate speech to the Greater Vancouver Regional Hospital District Board. As a result, they agreed to have the matter of Saint Mary's downgrading reconsidered by the board's hospital advisory committee. Mayor Evers was able to have that meeting take place two weeks later at Saint Mary's so that the members could see the hospital for themselves before voting. Although this effort to change the regional vote ultimately failed, the Greater Vancouver Regional Hospital

District did vote to look at using Saint Mary's for "non-acute programs."[73] Never shy of saying what he thought, Mayor Evers called the decision "a cop-out."[74] Delta Mayor Ernie Burnett, who chaired the committee, would comment later that the vote was based at least in part on the provincial government's requirement that the committee stay within a seven-hundred-bed limit for the area so that it was impossible for them to make a decision to approve Eagle Ridge as well as to keep Saint Mary's acute-care beds. Sister Mary Michael was infuriated and she pointed out that, even if Eagle Ridge were opened, there would still not be enough acute-care beds in the region.

In the meantime, it had been pointed out to Health Minister Mair that the report recommending the downgrading of Saint Mary's had only taken into account the patients coming to the hospital from New Westminster and Coquitlam but not those from Burnaby and Surrey and elsewhere in the province. Mair expressed surprise that the numbers had not been shown to him before, but he did not change his mind. He gave the hospital until October 31 to negotiate the terms for the conversion to extended care. The Saint Mary's forces seemed to be defeated.

Ultimately Saint Mary's was saved by providence. As the result of a cabinet shuffle, Jim Nielsen replaced Mair as Minister of Health, and everything was again up for grabs. In March 1981 Nielsen approved the construction of Eagle Ridge and announced that Saint Mary's would remain a full acute-care hospital, though of its 225 beds only 150 would now be used for acute care. But he also announced the development of upgraded laboratory and research facilities at Saint Mary's.

Mair's view on his successor's change of policy remains

unrepentant. "Nielsen screwed it up," he said in a 2005 interview. To his mind, it was logical to make Saint Mary's into a place for extended care. "Saint Mary's had found itself in the middle of an elderly demographic area, so it made sense to use it for that purpose. At that point, acute care could have been accommodated at other hospitals."[75] He never had any intention of closing Saint Mary's at the time. In fact, one of the reasons his government was considering Saint Mary's for extended care was because of its reputation for both medical and compassionate care services. Mair, who as Minister of Health had implemented the long-term care plan of his predecessor and introduced a home-care program, still feels strongly that government has failed on long-term care for seniors. "The NDP, the Liberals, every politician in that time needs to take some of the blame. . . . It is in abysmal shape now compared to what it ought to be. The baby boomers are here, and we're not ready for them. Every government since my time should take its share of the blame. Particularly in the Vander Zalm years and the NDP years it became an appalling crisis . . . Saint Mary's was a very fine hospital. Nobody made any criticism of it whatsoever. The decision was simply a technical decision based on where people needed help at that time."[76]

In 1982 the provincial government initiated a "restraint program," which meant massive cuts to hospital budgets, but because the announcement came when BC's hospitals were already one month into their fiscal year, they had no plans in place on how to handle the funding cuts. Thus, to implement cost cutting as quickly as possible, bed closures and layoffs were done on the fly. In April Saint Mary's closed twenty beds and laid off fifty-five full-time employees. Surrey Memorial Hospital was forced to begin planning bed closures even as they opened up a new fifth floor. Hospitals like Peace Arch that were already operating at over-capacity and taking only emergency patients balked at the cuts but were forced to cancel replacement staff for sick leave, vacations and resignations. Lions Gate Hospital laid off 144 people, about half of them nurses. The Vancouver General moved to eliminate six hundred staff positions. The Royal Inland Hospital at Kamloops announced the closure of eighty-four beds. Hospitals like Langley Memorial, which were already running deficits, were hit particularly hard because they were still being funded to serve smaller populations than they were actually serving in their rapidly growing areas. The desperate situation led them to begin charging a twenty-five dollar fee for some emergency procedures. But this was just the beginning, and any idea of new health programs in areas like long-term care had been slid onto the back burner by the government.

New Westminster MLA Dennis Cocke accused the government of closing twelve hundred beds around the province. In fact, almost 6 percent of the province's acute-care beds were ultimately closed. When the Hospital Employees Union called on hospital boards to stand up for patients and refuse to be compliant, some boards did so, perhaps sowing the seeds for the future regionalization of the system by politicians and bureaucrats who didn't like to be questioned or face opposition from people within the health-care system. Mayor Evers and the city council of New Westminster reacted angrily to the cuts but also to the government's management of the health-care system. The mayor demanded that the Health Minister explain why existing hospital beds were being closed even as the government was spending millions building or adding onto hospitals elsewhere. In June a meeting of two hundred doctors at Royal Columbian Hospital unanimously passed a motion calling on the hospital board to resign if they felt the hospital was not being funded adequately. Saint Mary's Hospital announced that close to one thousand people on its wait-lists for surgery would face further delays as the hospital struggled with the cutbacks.

Despite all the difficulties of these years, in 1986 Saint Mary's celebrated one hundred years of continuous service to New Westminster and British Columbians. It had survived typhoid and influenza epidemics, the Great Fire, the Great Depression and Rafe Mair. And although it had been badly affected by the provincial government "restraint program" in 1982–83 and the era of restricted funding that followed, forcing a reduction from 256 to 150 beds and the loss of both staff and services, the hospital had continued to develop its modern edge. Between 1983 and 1986 staff had decreased the time patients spent in hospital, increased outpatient services and strengthened the hospital's acute-care department. A rigorous standard of cleanliness had resulted in the lowest infection rate of all hospitals in the province. It had developed strong specialties in breast health, respiratory disease care, ophthalmology, and diabetic services and become a star teaching facility for its ear, nose and throat program. Though owned and operated by the Sisters of Providence, Saint Mary's was in effect governed by a community hospital board, funded by the provincial government, and a fully modern and integrated part of the provincial public health-care system. Its new corporate slogan was "A Tradition with a Future" and the mood was one of confidence and hope.

In 1986, after twenty-four years of dedicated service to the hospital and surrounding community, Sister Mary Michael retired as the administrator of Saint Mary's Hospital, and the board of trustees began their search for her successor. Although the Sisters of Providence proposed one of their order's novitiates, Mary Lei Gordon, for the position, she was not selected due to her lack of administrative experience in the health-care field. Instead, in a move that reflected a growing trend in Catholic hospitals across North America, the board chose to turn the administration over to non-clergy by selecting Bernie Bilodeau on the basis of his experience in the health-care field, particularly as the hospital's assistant administrator since 1975. Thus, he became the first lay administrator at Saint Mary's Hospital in its one hundred-year existence.

The change to a lay administration led to other changes in the hospital as management was moved from a centralized to a decentralized system of operation. Stephen Loader, finance director, and Elaine Sparks, nursing director, were promoted to assistant executive director positions in finance and nursing services, and in a move to make permanent the role of Saint Mary's as a cutting-edge hospital, Bilodeau added an assistant

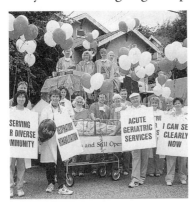

executive director for hospital planning and project management. Po Ang Yung, having a degree in health administration and extensive experience in hospital planning

Celebrating Saint Mary's. SAINT MARY'S HEALTH FOUNDATION.

and project management, was hired to meet this need. Each assistant executive director was given direct responsibility for a specific hospital department. Yet some old ways remained: the ever-frugal Saint Mary's filled these new positions with no increase to the hospital's administration budget.

By now it was apparent that if Saint Mary's was to remain as an acute-care hospital and solidify its programs and services, it would be necessary to improve its infrastructure. The first opportunity came as a result of an effort by three hospitals— Royal Columbian, Queens Park and Saint Mary's—to establish a palliative care unit at Saint Mary's. However, this million-dollar project also identified major problems in the hospital's heating and water supply system and brought to light the extensive amount of asbestos that existed in the structure. Rectifying these problems led to an expenditure of some $3 million over the next five years for asbestos removal, fire code and plumbing upgrade. Every area from the sub-basement to the seventh floor felt the impact, and it was amazing, if not miraculous, that throughout this period of renovation the hospital continued to carry the workload required to meet its budget commitments to the Ministry of Health. By 1993 all of these important projects were completed, as well as the upgrade of the air-handling system in the operating room and central supply department, improvements to the elevators, installation of a new phone system and hard-wiring for a centralized computer application. As a result, Saint Mary's entered the 1990s fully upgraded and renovated.

However, no sooner were the infrastructure upgrades completed, than the hospital received a $4.5 million approval to construct a new laboratory and pharmacy and an electrical vault, which would include emergency generators plus an additional space that would in later years become the centre for tuberculosis control for the Simon Fraser Health Region. The hospital's administration area and chapel on the ground floor areas were also renovated to become the Geriatric Day Hospital and the new home for the expanding Social Services Department. In 1992, the sixteen-bed palliative care unit was established for the North Fraser area and, by April 30, 1993, the Geriatric Day Hospital and twenty-five-bed Geriatric Assessment Unit were in full operation. These major projects, thanks to Po Ang Yung and plant director Russ Martin and his hard-working crew, were completed on time and on budget in January 1995. Not only was Saint Mary's active in upgrading its facility, it was also looking to solidify itself as a major player in the region for one-of-a-kind programs.

In the meantime, the Royal Columbian Hospital had been experiencing great difficulty in delivering services to hip-fracture patients, and in 1990 it was arranged that these patients would be transferred to Saint Mary's for their surgery, recovery and activation. This freed up Royal Columbian's busy emergency operating rooms and inpatient beds, which were being blocked for their incoming trauma patients. Saint Mary's initiative resulted in the establishment of an Activation Unit that could service not only hip-fracture patients but also other surgical in-patients, and it quickly became known throughout the North Fraser Region that Karen Van der Hoop, the director of Rehabilitation Services, and her well-trained staff ran a superb activation and rehabilitation department.

The central agency for the trustees of Saint Mary's Hospital was the British Columbia Health Association (BCHA), which had established seven area councils to elect the board members to the association. Saint Mary's was one of the hospitals in the BCHA's Fraser Valley Area Council, which covered the Fraser Valley from Hope to New Westminster, including Ladner. Saint Mary's administrator Bernie Bilodeau was the chair of the Fraser Valley Area Council, and from 1990 to 1995 he and Bonnie Anderson, chair of the Surrey Memorial Hospital board, were the two representatives for the Fraser Valley. He was also the chair of the BCHA's Human Resources Committee for five years and the chair of its Finance Committee in 1995. As a result, through his participation a number of opportunities became available to Saint Mary's. One of these was the Minis-

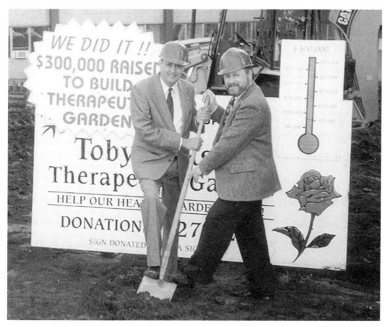

Breaking ground for the Toby Jackson Therapeutic Garden. Pictured are Paul Levy (left), chair of the hospital's foundation, and Rick Folka, chair of the hospital's board. SAINT MARY'S HEALTH FOUNDATION.

try of Health's pilot "Shared Governance for Nursing Practice" project, established in 1990. In a shared nursing structure, the responsibility, authority and accountability for practice decisions rests with the staff nurses, so this project established a number of practice councils that proved invaluable for addressing the many challenges in nursing practice at Saint Mary's. Shared Governance continued to be applied until Saint Mary's closed its doors in 2003.

In 1993 Saint Mary's had to meet a budget shortfall of 5 percent as the result of a "Health Accord" that was promoted by the NDP government. Finance Minister Glen Clark had negotiated a deal with three health-care unions and the agreement package included an estimated $50 million for wages and $20 million for early retirement as well as the reduction by 4,800 employees from the province's hospital workforce. This deal quickly proved to be much more costly than predicted and resulted in the closure of beds, a reduction in surgical services and, more importantly, the loss of young nurses and doctors who would be in great demand in the coming years.

However, the greatest change in health care in BC came in 1994 as an outcome of the 1991 "Closer to Home" report that Judge Peter Seaton of the BC Court of Appeal had prepared for the BC government. The basic message of his report was that health care in this province should be decentralized and that services should be brought closer to home. Underlying this proposal was the establishment of regional health boards and community health councils to which members or trustees would be elected every three years. These elected members would then be accountable to the community and not to the government. The new NDP government of Mike Harcourt responded in 1993 with a plan entitled "New Directions for a Healthy British Columbia," and in 1994 the Simon Fraser Health Region became the first health-care region in British Columbia. It included Maple Ridge, Coquitlam, Port Coquitlam, Port Moody and New Westminster (Burnaby was added in 1997) and covered an estimated 250,000 people. Initially the system maintained a degree of democratic representation because it was governed by a board that included representation from local Community Health Councils as well as from the city councils and school boards, who provided at least an indirect line of accountability to voters and served to protect the public trust on matters related to health care. Unfortunately, the provincial government had effective control through its appointed directors, which in the case of New Westminster included the former MLA Dennis Cocke.

All this seemed fine and in keeping with the rhetoric, but the running of health care had quietly become fundamentally different from the days when individuals could join hospital societies or when elected mayors and councillors served on regional hospital district boards. And there were other concerns. Buried in one Simon Fraser Health Region planning document was the note that "the Regional Health Board will be the sole employer for the region as a result of amalgamation of five health care societies." But no one at Saint Mary's Hospital had agreed to amalgamate and cease to be an employer. Was this a simple error or an inadvertent publication of the intentions of the government? It was then learned that those organizations that did not agree to allow the health region to be the employer faced the most unstable and worst possible funding arrangements—contracts.

To deal with this situation, some thirty-five religious groups and societies that owned hospitals or other health facilities and which, as part of their religious mission, had long provided health-care services in BC, formed a society called the Denominational Health Care Facilities Association. This new association developed a master agreement to ensure their rights to own, manage, operate and conduct the affairs of their respective facilities and to carry out their respective religious missions without undue interference or prejudice under the new system of appointed regional health authorities. The agreement, signed by Paul Ramsey, NDP Minister of Health, on March 16, 1995, stipulated that any religious organization that owned a health-care facility would, within four months of the execution of the master agreement, enter into an agreement with the local regional health authority. If there was no agreement within that time period, a panel would be appointed to advise the minister, for his or her sole discretion, to decide whether or not to terminate or initiate an affiliation agreement.

The board of trustees at Saint Mary's Hospital, trusting in the new process and the master agreement, struck a committee comprised of senior administration and board members. Although negotiations were difficult, the agreement, signed in May 1997 between the Simon Fraser Health Region and the Sisters of Charity of Providence in British Columbia did establish a requirement for proper notifications, the establishment of a panel with recommendations and a number of other procedures and safeguards. Since it was the first affiliation agreement signed by a denominational hospital in British Columbia, it became the template for other denominational facilities negotiating with their regional health authorities. The government would now retreat from some of its more draconian interventions in the affairs of non-profit societies, but its goal of greater control had been established.

In preparing for the advent of regionalization, in August 1995 the executive of the Saint Mary's board of trustees had passed a resolution that "given regionalization, regional alliances, the Denominational Facilities agreement and staff vacancies, the executive director evaluate the administrative structure and make recommendations to the board of trustees by February 20, 1996." This review was performed and a report submitted in October 1995, following which an ad hoc committee of the board, senior administration and hospital staff, along with Mike Mahoney from Health Management Resources as a facilitator, reviewed and made recommendations on the administrative structure at Saint Mary's. Mahoney's final report, submitted in May 1996, did not recommend any changes to the administrative structure but did identify concerns relating to the affiliation agreement with the region. His main emphasis, however, was on the new leadership role required to work with the region, to establish the hospital's role within the region relating to health care and non-negotiable services and programs. As well, he made recommendations for improvement in staff morale and in decision-making procedures and for a more secure place for Saint Mary's in the new health region. The board of trustees, as a result of the report and the administrative structure review, established a board committee to address the issues outlined in the report.

In October 1996 hospital head Bernie Bilodeau, after thirty-two years of excellent service overseeing the full modernization, renovation and development of the highly acclaimed specialized services at Saint Mary's, negotiated an early retirement effective February 28, 1997. Once again, the board began a search and in the early part of 1997 selected Hal Schmidt, formerly of Queen Alexandria Hospital in Victoria, as the hospital's new chief executive officer. Although officially already retired, Mr. Bilodeau continued until June 1, 1997, when Mr. Schmidt took over the helm.

Following Schmidt's hiring, Sister Mary Gordon, who had applied for the administrator's position in 1986, became a member of the Saint Mary's board. The board became concerned when she attempted to negotiate a private deal with the health authority without the board's knowledge or approval. She became visibly angry and distraught when confronted and insisted that her meetings with regional health officials were inconsequential, but she was not reappointed to the board the following year. Instead, she went on to become the treasurer for

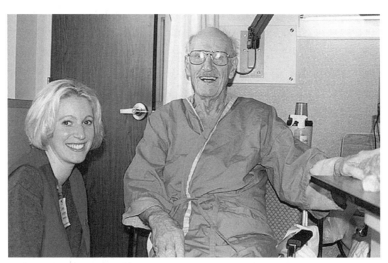

Saint Mary's staff were particularly known in the 1990s for their kind treatment of elderly patients. SAINT MARY'S HEALTH FOUNDATION.

the Sisters of Providence in BC, a position that would in the very near future allow her to affect financial matters relating to Saint Mary's in a most disastrous manner.

Over the ten-year period ending in March 1997, Saint Mary's Hospital had completed an estimated $10 million worth of major construction and infrastructure upgrades and the hospital now met all building-code requirements, including the seismic standards. During this time the hospital had also consolidated its core services in eye, ear, nose and throat care, rheumatology, respiratory rehabilitation and the pulmonary lab, the arthritis centre for the Simon Fraser Health Region, diagnostic mammography, geriatric day care, the geriatric assessment and treatment unit, the palliative care in-patient unit, and diabetic day care. The centres of excellence developed at Saint Mary's had become invaluable to the regional and provincial health-care system, receiving patients from throughout the Lower Mainland and British Columbia. Saint Mary's now also had a very active surgical role in support of its core programs in eye, ear, nose and throat and in breast cancer as well as hip and knee replacements and other surgical services. The hospital had a balanced budget and was thus in a good position to negotiate an affiliation agreement with the Simon Fraser Health Region with respect to its core and one-of-a-kind programs and services.

9

The Last Public Hospital

*"Democracy is the worst form of government. Except
for all of the other forms of government."*

—WINSTON CHURCHILL

HEALTH CARE IN BRITISH COLUMBIA had once been a model of democratic debate and representation. Hospitals were governed by societies whose annual general meetings were sometimes peaceful and sometimes battlegrounds over philosophic differences. Local politicians had input into the health-care system that served their communities and, while party loyalty had some influence on that input, having to face re-election and answer directly to voters in their own cities and municipalities generally proved to be a more powerful force. As a result, the provincial government's attempts to set province-wide policies had sometimes been frustrated, particularly when the government was seeking to implement cutbacks in health care.

Advocates of health-care regionalization routinely saw this

system as chaotic and inefficient. They knew that regionalization would be more efficient simply because it would dramatically reduce public involvement and the spread of information and debate, so they set out to sell the public and politicians on it with the vague promise of greater accountability in health care. However, as the health regions grew in size and power and large local bureaucracies came to increasingly dominate health care, it became more and more difficult for doctors and other health-care workers to speak out freely. At the same time all the expertise, local knowledge, deep concerns and community attachment of the hundreds of citizens who had volunteered their time and energy in the running of countless hospitals like Saint Mary's were cast aside and treated as of no value by the bureaucrats. In fact, this volunteerism had been the "oil" that kept the machinery running.

This change proved to be tragic for Saint Mary's and the thousands of patients who relied on the hospital. Saint Mary's became a hospital that was loved by a public that no longer had any representation in the health authority, even though it had been built and sustained through the will of that public. But while under regionalization Saint Mary's had become part of the provincial health system in all other ways, it was still an independent hospital with a community board. Unfortunately, independence was most unwelcome under the new regional system. It was seen as a relic of the days when there had been disagreement or even refusal to go along with the decisions made by the health-care bureaucracy in Victoria.

In 1998 the Simon Fraser Health Region, in keeping with the goals of the provincial government, decided to review all its hospitals to improve efficiency. The document that was produced, officially entitled "The Acute Care Review" but generally known as "The Hay Report" because the Hay Group from Ontario had been hired as consultants, concluded that it would be more efficient to have fewer hospitals—despite the fact that the population in the area was growing at an extremely rapid pace at the same time that it was aging.[77] The review also proposed that Saint Mary's Hospital become a "Primary Health Centre." In reality, the services this new primary health centre was to provide were not new at all but services such as rehabilitation and palliative care for which Saint Mary's was already well known. However, in the new model, Saint Mary's would no longer offer acute-care services, and surgery would be moved to hospitals such as Eagle Ridge. Once again the government was suggesting that removing surgical services from the most efficient hospital in the region would somehow reduce the pressure on the Royal Columbian Hospital.

Saint Mary's Hospital used its independence to fight the recommendations, and doctors, patients and the public openly rebelled. Leading the fight behind the scenes was Hal Schmidt who had become CEO of Saint Mary's in 1997. He had been one of twelve administrators on the Acute Care Review committee and the only one representing an independent hospital not controlled by the health authority, and he soon realized that the review was not friendly and the focus was only on saving money. It took just a few meetings before recommendations to reduce the role of Saint Mary's Hospital were brought forward, and at one point Schmidt was told by an official that "there is no role for religion in health care."[78] (At this point there were thirteen religious organizations and twenty-five non-profit groups in BC operating thirty-eight health-care facilities, employing approximately ten thousand people and operating almost 14,800 beds.) Schmidt began to understand the extent of the tension between the Simon Fraser Health Region and Saint Mary's Hospital when one executive at the health authority asked him why he took the job at Saint Mary's if he was just there to close the hospital, and he recognized that this unhealthy attitude was shared by a number of the other officials. He put this down to the health authority's unofficial operating credo of "if we don't own it and control it, we don't want it."[79] He also gained the impression that although "Saint Mary's and Royal Columbian worked as a team in terms of health care," they did not seem to like each other.

When the region had proposed reviewing costs in acute care, Schmidt's first thoughts were, "anything we can do to rationalize costs and deliver better services would be great." However, he soon learned that under the new funding arrangements

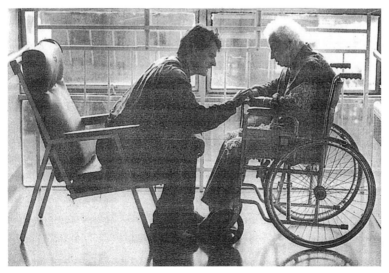

Physiotherapist with elderly patient. *THE RECORD*, OCTOBER 3, 1993, P. 11.

Saint Mary's would face a serious budget shortfall. His own analysis told him that Saint Mary's was already shortchanged when it came to funding: while health authority budgets had increased by 24.7 percent over the last five years, funding to Saint Mary's had only increased by 8.6 percent when it really needed an estimated 17 percent to 19 percent to maintain the status quo. Despite this, Saint Mary's had managed to deliver services while decreasing costs each year and increasing operating-room time.

As Schmidt sought to protect Saint Mary's, it became apparent that health officials saw him as a renegade, not a team player in their new health-care system. Realizing that this was an obstacle to working in the new system of regional bureaucracies, he decided that the hospital could not live simply on its history and the quality of its work, and he implemented a strategic planning process, one in which the hospital would proactively participate as part of a regional health-care system.

Officially the purpose of the review of acute care had been to improve efficiency, although nowhere does the document identify what would be more efficient about the plan or how the primary issue of efficiency in hospitals and long waiting lists for surgery would be addressed. Perhaps the answer lies in the "Financial Considerations" part of the report, which states that the resulting "savings" from the proposed restructuring would be approximately $14 million. This is less than the 10 percent that the government had set as its goal for reducing the budget for acute hospital care in the region but greater than the 5 percent identified as a minimum goal. However, the report contained some big assumptions when it came to cost saving, including the idea that the number of days people spend in hospital should be substantially reduced. For example, it was assumed, without actually testing it first, that hospital stays for newborns could be reduced by 15 percent and that sending more people home immediately after operations could reduce hospital stays by 25 percent. Another part of the government's plan was to reduce by 90 percent the number of days patients spent in hospital while awaiting transfer to nursing homes or other long-term care facilities, but other than a general statement about increasing home-care services, it was unclear where the ten thousand affected patients would go. In fact, if hospital beds were freed up in this way, they would most likely be used for persons on the surgery waiting lists. But while the use of more beds for more operations would be efficient in the old sense of treating more patients, it would be inefficient when it came to saving money. More surgeries would actually cost the health authority more.

When the final report was issued in August 1998, Schmidt and the Saint Mary's board knew that it was flawed. However, his view of the Simon Fraser Health Region board was that it was made up of people who, lacking any experience in health care, were forced to rely on health-authority administrators for decision-making information. He therefore hoped that, by presenting good information to the board on the importance of maintaining Saint Mary's as an acute-care hospital, he could overcome the recommendations of the Acute Care Review.

In September 1998 the war over the future of health care in the region heated up, and it looked like the battle over the future of Saint Mary's Hospital might become more a defence of health care in general. When the government released a report on palliative care, a group of palliative care nurses that included Bev Welsh from Saint Mary's Hospital had this to say:

> Palliative care is active, compassionate care of the terminally ill at a time when their disease is no longer responsive to traditional treatment for cure or prolongation of life, and when the control of symptoms—physical, emotional and spiritual—is paramount. This care is delivered in an acute hospital setting . . . The proposed reduction of acute (in-hospital) palliative beds from thirty-four to twelve in a region servicing a population of 650,000 is inadequate . . . If Saint Mary's is stripped of its acute-care services as the Hay Group recommends, the acute palliative care unit in the region will be under-supported. If you are unable to continue caring for your loved one at home, with reduced palliative beds, where will you go? . . . The proposed residential hospices would provide comfort rather than active treatment to patients while supporting members through a time of illness, death, and bereavement . . . Families caring for critically ill palliative patients at home may be burdened with the expense of costly medications and medical supplies. (Costs currently range from hundreds to thousands of dollars monthly.) All terminally ill have the right to quality of life at the end of life.

The fight was now on and the government took a beating in the media. Even the Sisters of Providence, who owned the hospital, decided to fight back and took the unprecedented step of going public. In a media release, Sister Betty Kaczmarczyk said that "the Sisters of Charity of Providence in BC, owners and operators of Saint Mary's Hospital in New Westminster for the past

112 years, have labeled a consultant's report that recommends removal of the hospital's acute-care status as a seriously flawed document."[80] In the same release, Rick Folka, chairman of the hospital board, said, "We see no real benefits to the people of the Health Region in eliminating all acute care services currently provided by Saint Mary's Hospital. We are confident that the Simon Fraser Health Board and administration will also recognize that their endorsement of the acute care recommendations will create an unnecessary hardship for people within the Region."[81] Doctors also opposed the recommendations, and among them were many who did not practise at Saint Mary's. Doctor Bob Hayden, president of the medical staff at Royal Columbian Hospital, told the media that "everything we hear speaks about the fact you will have to do more with less, more with less and more with less. But be careful, because you can chant that mantra until it becomes 'more with nothing.'"[82]

The BC government tried to defend itself by arguing that the federal government's downloading of health-care costs was putting a strain on the province and that BC was providing a higher level of funding than other provinces. But the public backlash was focused on the local effects, and as a result the planned downgrading of Saint Mary's emerged as the most controversial health issue in the province and became a symbol of the public's concern, because it looked more and more like an attempt to loot the resources of the region's last independent and publicly governed hospital than an attempt to promote efficiency. To many people it seemed to be putting the cart before the horse that, with four thousand people in the region already on wait-lists for surgery, the government would close Saint Mary's seven operating rooms on the vague promise that the system would be more efficient sometime in the future. In fact, Saint Mary's was renowned for its efficiency, having bumped only one patient from scheduled surgery in eighteen years. The hospital did more eye surgeries than all the other hospitals in the region combined, more than three times the number done at Burnaby Hospital, which was supposed to take over much of the work of Saint Mary's. With its efficiency and lower costs, it made more sense for Saint Mary's to be doing more surgery in the region, not less.

A group of prominent citizens that included Michael Crean, Janis Fiolleau, J. Glenn Gates, Paul Levy, Del Patterson, Dr. Hugh Parsons, Irene Petruk, Pat Philley and Mary Strzelecki formed "The Friends of Saint Mary's Hospital" and announced that they were "deeply concerned with the recommendations of the Simon Fraser Health Region's Acute Care Review and the shattering impact it would have on Saint Mary's Hospital in providing valuable acute-care services to the residents of New Westminster and the broader Simon Fraser Health Region."[83] New Westminster City Council once again became involved and provided outright support for the Friends as did the City of Burnaby. Adding to the pressure was the organized and vocal opposition of the Catholic Church, with priests speaking on the matter from their pulpits, urging support for the Friends. And then there were the petitions. On September 17 senior citizens Irene Petruk and Anne Kroeker delivered a 750-page petition to health authority CEO Jim Fair. It contained sixteen thousand signatures opposed to the proposed changes, and the fiery Petruk made it clear that the effort would not stop there. "We're not done yet,"[84] she vowed. The petition eventually had over twenty-two thousand signatures.

In an attempt to calm the waters, the Simon Fraser Health Board called an "information meeting" for September 23, 1998, but the Friends of Saint Mary's reacted quickly by organizing a protest march to the event. This meeting was critical. There had to be a strong showing of support and the group hoped to fill the 110-seat meeting room in the city library that health officials had booked for the occasion. Paul Levy, the chair of the hospital's foundation, emerged as the key spokesperson for the group and assertively replied to any attempt to denigrate their motives. When the public was accused of being opposed to change, Levy pointed out just how much Saint Mary's had changed over the past one hundred years. He warned the region not to try to address problems in health care through "change just for the sake of change."[85]

The impasse between Saint Mary's and the health region had now reached the point that there could not even be agreement on the choice of the meeting room. When the Friends of Saint Mary's and the local newspaper, *The Record*, urged the region to hold the meeting in a larger space to be sure of accommodating all who wished to attend, Helen Carkner, spokesperson for the Region replied, "We wanted the community to talk without too large a crowd." Accusing the Friends of organizing a protest, she went on to say, "New Westminster is being mobilized and there is a push to get people out." If people wanted to come to the meeting to protest, she said, "they'll be doing that outside."[86]

On the day of the meeting, protesters marched throughout the normally quiet city. If the health-care system had come to resemble feudal baronies, the marchers looked like a ragtag army of ancient rebels. Led by bagpiper Bill Sneddon as if marching out to battle, they looked as if a whole village had risen up against its oppressors. Women in their seventies and older were joined by a Catholic priest and city councillors. Banners flew, speeches were given and picket signs were waved in the air by people who were probably more accustomed to holding teas for the hospital than protesting against government. And just like the rebels of old, most of them would not be welcomed into the castle. When the meeting room was full, a sign was placed on the elevator, a cordon of police officers stood guard, and more than two hundred people were forced to remain outside. The anger was palpable, and the non-stop chanting and the wailing bagpipes could easily be heard in the basement meeting room. *The Record* accused the health region of nearly starting a "mini-riot."[87]

But while they may have locked out two hundred of the three hundred protesters, health officials also found themselves locked in the library where Simon Fraser Health Region Board chair Dennis Cocke, CEO James Fair and vice-president of acute services Joanne Konnert faced an onslaught of anger and frustration but also thoughtful debate and opinion. Irene Petruk, the first person to the microphone, immediately rose to the support of those locked out. "Why in heaven's name conduct a meeting of this magnitude and importance to citizens of this area in a hall that holds barely a hundred?" she asked.[88] When Konnert told the assembly that Saint Mary's equipment would be moved to other hospitals, it created a prolonged and angry outburst in a city that knew full well that much of the equipment had been paid for by the local community. One senior, Burnaby resident Joan Curle, who could barely see for herself while she waited for eye surgery, presented a petition of five thousand signatures that she had collected. Doctor Rob

Irvine attacked the report that had brought about the crisis for criticizing the appearance of Saint Mary's Hospital by saying, "It's like people. It's what goes on inside that counts."[89]

Finally the Health Board agreed to hold a second public meeting in a larger space on September 30. Immediately, the Friends of Saint Mary's were faced with a serious challenge because the board had deliberately scheduled it for the largest possible meeting space in the city, the twelve hundred-seat Massey Theatre. The Friends knew that with just three hundred protesters in that large theatre the room would look nearly empty and that this would create the wrong impression on the evening television newscasts. They also knew that the health region was gambling that the protesters could not possibly fill the hall, so with just one week to organize before the meeting, the Friends of Saint Mary's had their work cut out for them. However, the support was out there; hospital CEO Hal Schmidt was getting phone calls from 6:00 a.m. to past midnight as people tried to get through to express their support for the hospital.

On the appointed day the theatre was full and the lobby was packed. *Record* reporter Lori Pappajohn would write: "Standing ovations, thunderous applause, cheers, heckles and boos filled Massey Theatre Wednesday night as twelve hundred people packed the theatre to defend Saint Mary's Hospital."[90] It was the most democratic participation that the health-care system in the region had seen in years. Doctor Rudy Weitemeyer told the crowd that the consultants who had written the report recommending the end of Saint Mary's acute-care status had only spent fifteen minutes inside the hospital. Joan Curle, who had collected five thousand signatures on a petition just a week earlier, announced that she had gathered another four thousand since that time. Paul Levy asked how the government "could be so out of touch with the people,"[91] and when Catholic Archbishop Adam Exner took the floor to condemn the decision in an eloquent speech, the crowd roared its approval. He told them that singling out Saint Mary's struck at the root of freedom of religion. Of particular concern to him was the loss of pastoral care as a part of acute care in the region and its importance as part of health care. The Archbishop's speech drew a long and rousing standing ovation.

"While this was going on inside, I saw a nurse in tears standing in the theatre lobby," reported Karl Crosby, the hospital's head of public relations. "When I asked her why she was crying, she responded, 'I had no idea that so many people cared about us [Saint Mary's].'" Now the fight was underway in earnest and Saint Mary's, hoping that the board would see the flawed assumptions in the report, prepared a response for the regional board's November meeting. They had little doubt that the new system of regionalization had more to do with saving money than it did with delivery of better health care. After all, Saint Mary's had performed more than thirteen thousand operations the year before, and in some areas such as breast health Saint Mary's was the leader for the entire region.

By November the health-care system in the region was facing a rebellion of its own employees, and the planned weekend meeting of the Simon Fraser Health Region board was cancelled after the BC Nurses Union said that it would impose a ban on overtime for nurses if the meeting went ahead. In December a reporter with *Burnaby Now*, Dan Hilborn, revealed that the region's board had become sharply divided over the Acute Care Review and its proposed downgrading of Saint Mary's Hospital. Board member Mike Milaney expressed his own lack of confidence in the handling of the matter by the region's administrators when he said, "Frankly, the sooner we bury this report the better . . . To me, nobody in this room from administration or the board can give their [Saint Mary's] side of the story . . . We're talking about closing down the acute care service of an institution that's been around for 110 years."[92] Helene Greenaway, the BC Nurses Union representative on the board, urged the board to "respect the views of citizens expressed at recent public meetings."[93]

The day after Hilborn's article appeared, it was announced at a press conference that no change to Saint Mary's Hospital would occur until there was consultation with the hospital's representatives. The matter was now out of the hands of the administrators of the Simon Fraser Health Region, and future negotiations would be handled by Dennis Cocke, the board chair of the Simon Fraser Health Region. In January 1999 he announced that a formal agreement had been reached with Saint Mary's Hospital. In something of an understatement, he acknowledged, "As you all know, following the release of the Hay Report and its recommendations, the board received a considerable amount of feedback from residents of our communities, staff, physicians and many others." He said he wanted to change health care in the region to deal with the growing population and to reduce costs, but he also wanted to respect public opinion and to avoid damaging health care in the process. The agreement, he said, was "a win-win for both of us,"[94] and in some ways it was the best of both worlds. Saint Mary's would do much of the rehabilitation and care for the elderly and enhanced breast health that the government was seeking, and Cocke would ultimately agree not to close the hospital's operating rooms. Saint Mary's would do general surgery and keep its centres of excellence in ophthalmology, ear, nose and throat. Saint Mary's would also relieve some of the pressure on Royal Columbian Hospital by caring for some patients after surgery and freeing up beds in that hospital's emergency department. What's more, "and to me this is one of the most exciting aspects of the agreement," said Cocke, "Saint Mary's Hospital will become the region's centre for specialized rehabilitation."[95] At this time 60 percent of the region's residents requiring specialized rehabilitation (cardiac, neuro, respiratory and post-trauma) had to go outside of the region and often had to endure long waits. Plans were still being made to move some surgery to Eagle Ridge Hospital, but Cocke and his board had now acknowledged and entrenched the value and efficiency of Saint Mary's surgical programs.

Schmidt welcomed the agreement and looked forward to the hospital's new role in developing the best rehabilitation program possible for its patients. It seemed once again that Saint Mary's was saved and facing a bright future, but there was some concern at the hospital that the region's bureaucrats might not honour the agreement made by their governing board and, as a precaution, the hospital's officials asked that the agreement be put in writing. Meanwhile, the board of the Simon Fraser Health Region had once again turned the matter over to its administrative staff, but they were definitely not happy, and when an implementation committee was struck between the region and Saint Mary's, it quickly became clear that there were different interpretations of the agreement. The region's representatives wanted those parts of it that favoured the

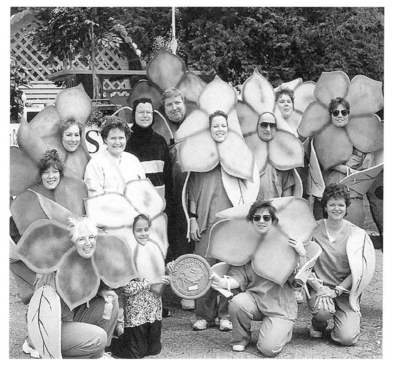

Saint Mary's staff often participated in events to reach out to the community. SAINT MARY'S HEALTH FOUNDATION.

region to be implemented immediately. These included such things as the closing of beds at Saint Mary's, which would have resulted in immediate loss of funding to the hospital and immediate savings to the Simon Fraser Health Region. Schmidt took the position that removal of any programs had to coincide with the promised expansion. When the health region wanted Saint Mary's to close its intensive-care unit, which was needed to support its ear, nose and throat surgical program, their disagreements reached an impasse.

On April 20, 2000, the hospital's board chair John

Michalski wrote a letter to new Simon Fraser board chair Paul McDonnell to say that Saint Mary's would not participate in implementation of the agreement as interpreted by the health authority administration. "In fact," wrote Michalski, "the process appears to be nothing more than a marginalization and downsizing of Saint Mary's Hospital to validate upsizing Eagle Ridge Hospital at a significant financial cost and organizational upheaval."[96] Following Michalski's letter, Schmidt and Michalski met with the provincial Minister of Health, Mike Farnsworth. No details of the meeting were revealed, but Schmidt believes that Farnsworth had intervened behind the scenes in support of Saint Mary's. While the appeal to the minister may have angered health region officials, the hospital had simply used what was left of the democratic process in health care, appealing to the only person with elected office in the province who still had any direct influence over local health care.

Facing a direct confrontation with the health region's powerful bureaucracy, the hospital's supporters knew they were in a race against time. On May 6 an extraordinary meeting was held between the board of trustees of Saint Mary's Hospital and the executive council of the Sisters of Charity of Providence in British Columbia; the result was the passage of a motion to seek expedited mediation. Doctor John G. Wade and Claude R. Thomson, QC, were selected as the arbitration panel. The view at Saint Mary's was that the health region's submission to the arbitrators lacked research and that this would be evident in their presentation; this was proved true when just three and half days into the arbitration process the Simon Fraser Health Region notified the arbitrator that they had no idea the two parties were so far apart and that they would not be returning to the table. In an unprecedented display of arrogance and bad faith, they had reneged on the binding arbitration called for in the agreement they had signed just four months earlier. All the months of discussion, a written agreement and the intervention of the region's board and even the involvement of the Minister of Health were for nothing, and Saint Mary's found itself back in the position it had been in three years earlier—vulnerable and alone in a system that was determined to cut costs and sacrifice Saint Mary's to do it. The government could have ordered the implementation of the agreement at any time if they had so wished, but by this time the NDP government was facing an impending election and almost certain defeat, making any further appeal to the region's board or the minister largely irrelevant.

The May 2001 election saw a crushing defeat for the NDP. The Liberal Party of British Columbia took all but two seats in the provincial legislature and Gordon Campbell became the new premier. By this time the battle to keep Saint Mary's as an acute-care hospital under the new system of unelected regional health authorities had dragged on for four long years without resolution, but there was great hope at Saint Mary's that the new government would support the hospital. After all, while in Opposition the Liberals had raked the NDP over the coals when their government had closed Shaughnessy Hospital. Liberal health critic Linda Reid had said of that hospital's closure at a "Save Shaughnessy" rally, "This is the last straw!"[97] The BC Medical Association and the BC Nurses Union had been publicly criticizing the government over health care. In New Westminster, soon-to-be-elected Liberal Joyce Murray had been a strong participant in the movement to keep Saint Mary's as an acute-care hospital and had been a vocal critic of the government on the issue, earning the support of many of the hospital's proponents. The Liberals had made improved health care a central plank of their campaign platform and promised that there would be no more hospital closures.

However, the new government moved quickly to put its own stamp on the health-care system, and by December had created new and even larger health authorities by reducing the number of regions from fifty-two to just five. All remnants of any elected representation with elected officials were gone, and the local community health councils were abolished. When it came to assessing health-care needs in a community or even a neighbourhood, New Westminster was now linked with Delta, Coquitlam with Chilliwack, and Burnaby with Hope and Boston Bar in the new Fraser Health Authority. These new regions made health care in British Columbia less local than it had ever been in the province's history. Officially health care would now be in the hands of "local" health authorities, but in reality the directors would be appointed exclusively by the provincial government. Independent hospitals like Saint Mary's found themselves facing monumentally powerful health-care authorities, which no longer had to deal with any locally elected mayors or city councillors. The history of health authorities, and particularly the reforms instituted by the Liberals, is a chilling example of the ease with which democratic forms of government can be dispensed.

There was one other change to the health authorities under the new government. For the first time, health authority board members would be paid for sitting on a board. Individual board members of the Fraser Health Authority were paid

$7,500 per year while the new board chair, Barry Forbes, was to be paid $15,000. Across British Columbia the cost of paying the small group of fifty-four people selected by the provincial government to sit on health authority boards was $450,000. This money was paid whether or not a board member actually attended meetings, but each member also netted an additional $500 for every board and committee meeting at which he actually appeared. Should board members be required to attend any other meetings, they would be paid an extra $250. Should half a dozen board members of the Fraser Health Authority decide to meet citizens upset over the closure of Saint Mary's Hospital, even that small number would receive $3,000 just for showing up. Prior to this, these had been volunteer positions. All this occurred when the board's budget had increased by 25 percent while the number of patients served had fallen by 5 percent and waiting lists had grown dramatically, up to 89 percent in some cases.

A former board member of the Simon Fraser Health Board, Helene Greenaway, publicly commented that as a volunteer she had no one to answer to but the public she served and wondered if things would change. "We're not talking about a board of community stakeholders anymore. We're talking a board that has to run a business-like operation," responded Elizabeth Watson, managing director of board resourcing and development for the provincial government.[98] It is interesting to note that not a single member of a health region board has ever spoken out against the provincial government since these payments were implemented.

The new health authority board chair, Barry Forbes, had been well known in New Westminster as the CEO of

Westminster Credit Union and for his involvement with Douglas College, Burnaby Hospital and the New Westminster Chamber of Commerce. At Saint Mary's his appointment inspired high hopes that the new regime would lead to positive developments, and Forbes and his administration became the targets of Saint Mary's advocates hoping to establish a new and more positive relationship, particularly in light of the Liberals' election promises on health care. The hospital had been in a vacuum for months. However, their overtures were greeted by silence at the official level. But the bureaucrats were not silent, and at one point it was suggested to Schmidt that he might take over Eagle Ridge Hospital and that Eagle Ridge could then become the new Saint Mary's. Another official suggested that matters could be resolved if Schmidt had two masters, perhaps becoming a minor official at Saint Mary's but a vice-president within the health authority. These attempts to win his loyalty were presented mostly as casual remarks—as if the health authority was testing his resolve to defend Saint Mary's.

When Bob Smith was hired as the CEO for the Fraser Health Authority, Schmidt saw an opportunity to forge a new relationship. It seemed to him that the change in government and structure had created fertile ground for Saint Mary's Hospital, so when Smith asked Schmidt and hospital board chair Betty Wynne for a meeting on his first day on the job, Saint Mary's hospital representatives were delighted. Schmidt was sure that Smith wanted to tie up loose ends and resolve the now long-running dispute between the health authority and Saint Mary's. However, it was unusual to invite a board chair from a hospital to a meeting without knowing what it was about, so Schmidt asked Smith for a meeting alone in the morning to determine its purpose. That is when Smith told him that the Fraser Health Authority would be terminating its agreement with Saint Mary's Hospital. Schmidt protested that the hospital provided valuable health care and offered solutions, but he was told simply that not everybody gets what they want. When the afternoon meeting was held, hospital board chair Betty Wynne made it clear to Smith that cutting off all funding to Saint Mary's would not be the end of the matter.

Following the meeting with Smith, Fraser Health Chair Forbes advised the administration at Saint Mary's that the FHA board had supported the cancellation of the affiliation agreement. According to Schmidt, Forbes scolded him and Wynne, telling them that they should have seen it coming, and that health authority officials had provided warning. Schmidt insists that no such warning had been given—not that it would have justified the sudden decision taken by the health authority. He describes the tone of the meetings with Forbes and Smith as "arrogant and mean-spirited."[99]

Everyone at Saint Mary's was genuinely surprised by the disastrous turn of events, but Schmidt knew that the hospital's campaign against downgrading had earned bitter enmity from some officials in the health authority and from the provincial Ministry of Health, which had become tired of the political headache known as Saint Mary's Hospital. Speculation on how the decision had come about in the increasingly closed circle of health-care administration in BC was rife at Saint Mary's and among the public, but given the newness of Forbes and Smith to their roles, it was generally accepted that there were only two possibilities: it was either based on what they were told from inside the FHA or on what they were ordered to do from Victoria. In reality, it was a combination of both.

In fact, the Fraser Health Authority had produced an internal report in late February 2002, after only a couple of months of existence, recommending the closure of Saint Mary's Hospital. The following month a second internal report authored by the health authority and recommending the hospital's closure was sent to the Minister of Health Services. But on April 25, 2002, when the Fraser Health Authority had announced its Clinical Services Directional Plan, there had been no mention of reducing funding or closing Saint Mary's Hospital. Instead, there was the usual suggestion of greater efficiency and consolidation of services between Saint Mary's and Eagle Ridge. The Saint Mary's board had responded by requesting a joint meeting between the hospital board and the regional board for clarification. There was no response. In early May 2002, after months of secret planning, the health authority had prepared its final internal report recommending the full closure of Saint Mary's Hospital. There had been no public awareness of these secret proceedings and no consultation with the Sisters of Providence or the hospital board and administration.

In the meantime, Schmidt had accepted a position with Providence Health Care, an umbrella group of Catholic hospitals that did not include Saint Mary's, but he had agreed to remain on as Saint Mary's CEO until a replacement was found. On June 24 Schmidt was informed by the health authority that Saint Mary's would no longer receive funding from the provincial government. In a meeting with the health authority's CEO Smith, Schmidt and the hospital's board members learned that the termination of the hospital's affiliation agreement with the health authority would result in the loss of 93 percent of the hospital's budget. Smith was emphatic that the region's funding shortfall of $126 million required the closure of a facility because it would help to fill the underused Eagle Ridge Hospital. When asked if any other hospitals were to be treated in the same way, the Saint Mary's representatives were told that there would be major impacts at Hope, Mission and Delta. Then Smith made it clear that he intended to move quickly on the closure of Saint Mary's.

However, in their eagerness to get rid of the hospital, the health authority had overlooked the fact that the provincial master agreement with denominational (religious) health-care facilities required consultation before critical changes could be made to any affiliated hospital. The health authority, therefore, backed off, and on July 10 Forbes delivered a letter to the hospital giving notice of termination of the affiliation agreement in one year as required by its terms. Closure of the hospital was now scheduled for July 10, 2003, and this time it looked like there was no stopping the forces allied against Saint Mary's.

Some holidays were cancelled at Saint Mary's in the summer of 2002 as staff prepared arguments for a review panel that was to determine the legality of the health authority's decision to end its affiliation agreement with the hospital. This time the authority's officials could not simply walk away and shut down the process as they had with the arbitration in 2000. But it would take months for the panel to come to its final conclusions and once again the Friends of Saint Mary's were active, this time to fight for the institution's very existence. But Schmidt realized that, even if Saint Mary's won the right to remain open, the hostility toward the hospital was deeply and permanently entrenched at the health authority. There needed to be some other solution. He suggested a merger between Saint Mary's and the Providence Group as an option that would remove Saint Mary's from the control of the Fraser Health Authority and still give it a role as an acute-care facility.

He took this concept to the headquarters of the Sisters of Providence in Montreal where, according to Schmidt, the Sisters wanted to know what they could expect financially in return. He replied that the benefit would be in saving the hospital and continuing its mission of compassionate health care started over one hundred years earlier. The institutions that had combined to form Providence Health Care had received no money to carry out this mandate in the past. In an interview in 2005, Schmidt said, "By now, we were looking to Providence as our lifeline. And we were saying we want money from them to save us."[100]

But not all the Sisters or even the members of the hospital board agreed with Schmidt. Some still optimistically believed the panel findings would support the hospital. The Friends of Saint Mary's decided to open the fall with a large gamble—to hold its own rally and once again fill the twelve hundred-seat Massey Theatre, and the long notice period allowed hospital advocates two months to organize for the important date. The city was once again united and at this time Liberal MLA Joyce Murray publicly supported the hospital. The gamble paid off when the theatre was completely filled, making it the largest public protest in the history of New Westminster, but neither Health Board Chair Forbes nor Fraser Health Authority CEO Smith attended, though they had been invited to do so. Board Chair Betty Wynne told the crowd that Saint Mary's had "something to teach the rest of them. We're effective, efficient and compassionate."[101] Archbishop Adam Exner spoke out against the government's actions. Once again, the opposition to tampering with the status of Saint Mary's Hospital was threatening the popularity of a government, only this time the stakes were much higher and the supporters of Saint Mary's were that much more determined.

Throughout the following months the campaign to save the hospital gathered strength, and the health authority came to regret the year-long notice of closure. October saw local Member of Parliament Paul Forseth publicly denounce Premier Gordon Campbell, insisting that the decision to close Saint Mary's had always been a done deal and must have been approved at the very top. The stakes were raised again when protesters against the planned closure of the emergency department at Delta Hospital formed a coalition and demonstrated at a health authority board meeting. By the third week of October, New Westminster and vicinity was home to three thousand lawn signs bearing the slogan, "Still Serving, Worth Saving." In November, MLA Murray held a "Dialogue on Saint Mary's," essentially requiring health authorities to face medical advisors, church representatives, the Friends of Saint Mary's and a couple of community members. Both Forbes and Smith appeared, although reluctantly. They seemed little interested in the proceedings, had little to say and spent part of the meeting on their cellphones. They made no response to any points made by the presenters. Petitions were circulated again and this time the effort was run out of city hall itself. So many petitions landed so quickly on the desk of Mayor Helen Sparkes that a large box had to be used to hold them all. More than twenty thousand signatures were presented to the legislature in Victoria.

Meanwhile, even as the government was attempting to close Saint Mary's, the hospital kept winning awards for its excellence, including the full endorsement of the business community. Betty Wynne accepted an award from the Chamber of Commerce as Saint Mary's won the "large business of the year" award. *BC Business* magazine placed Saint Mary's on its "A-list," ranking it number thirteen on its list of the top twenty-five best employers in BC. Schmidt was presented with the Performance Citation Award of the Catholic Health Association in Canada, the highest award in Catholic health care.

In January 2003 the panel ruled in favour of Saint Mary's Hospital. *The Province* newspaper described the decision as "a stay of execution."[102] The panel was damning in its assessment

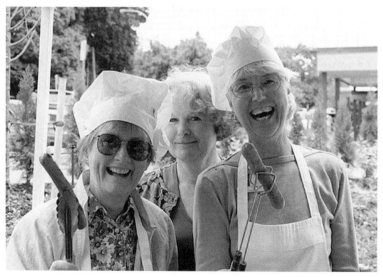

The last chair of the Saint Mary's Hospital Board, Betty Wynne on the left, at a hospital event. SAINT MARY'S HEALTH FOUNDATION.

of the Fraser Health Authority, ruling that the FHA had failed to give proper consideration to the hospital's own money-saving proposals—the Saint Mary's plan would have actually saved more than the $17.2 million that the FHA would save by closing the hospital—and it described Saint Mary's as an invaluable pressure release for the overcrowded Royal Columbian Hospital. "The FHA clearly made a determination not to consult with Saint Mary's as part of its deliberations. We are frankly quite surprised," said panel chair Donald Munroe. And confident that they had a future once more, Saint Mary's hired Larry Odegard as the new CEO of the hospital.

10

The Last Betrayal

"When you murder a person, you go to jail. What happens when you kill a hospital?"

—A SUPPORTER OF SAINT MARY'S HOSPITAL

FROM JANUARY TO APRIL 2003 Saint Mary's Hospital and the Fraser Health Authority worked behind the scenes to resolve their differences, and on April 15, 2003, FHA CEO Bob Smith and Saint Mary's new hospital CEO Larry Odegard held a news conference to announce that an agreement had been reached that guaranteed Saint Mary's remained open as an acute-care hospital. The news made the headlines. "Saint Mary's gets a new deal,"[103] *The Record* announced. "Beloved New West Hospital survives with new role,"[104] *The Vancouver Sun* trumpeted. ⁓ 1 the mood throughout the city and surrounding ⁣es was one of celebration. It seemed once again that ⁣ninistry had recognized the value of the hospital ⁣ry's would still have a long-term role within the ⁣ authority. But here and there a reporter would ask how much funding Saint Mary's would receive under the new deal. Each time, there was no clear answer.

The Fraser Health Authority and Saint Mary's agreed to a fifteen-month transition period for the new plan to be implemented, and the health authority and hospital's senior management began to work out the details of the new role that Saint Mary's would play within the region. A few points were already clear. Saint Mary's would now be under a purchaser/provider relationship with the FHA, meaning that it would be selling health care to the government rather than have its own guaranteed funding like other hospitals in British Columbia. What the public did not know was that under the new arrangement, Saint Mary's would lose two-thirds of its funding or roughly $20 million annually. The government would provide only $11.85 million. To maintain its programs, Saint Mary's would have to find new funding from other sources through contracts or partnerships with private health-care companies. While Health Authority CEO Bob Smith was telling the public that the FHA was now championing the mission of Saint Mary's Hospital, in reality, the government was telling Saint Mary's that it could remain open, but it would be up to the hospital to sort out exactly how to do that with minimal public funding. The health authority had effectively ended the public outcry and media storm by misleading everyone into believing that Saint Mary's would continue to serve the thousands of patients who had come to depend on its special level of care. In reality the new deal was no deal at all. The only people outside the authority who were aware of this reality were the region's MLAs and their assistants who were assembled on September 10, 2003, at the Sherbrooke Centre in New Westminster to be given the exact dates and amounts of the phased cuts. This would have been a fine opportunity for one of them to speak out, but none of them did. The MLAs were also told that the FHA's share of the health deficit of $105 million was to be $29 million spread over three years, but that the overwhelming portion of that would be garnered by the cut to Saint Mary's funding. The two top goals of the FHA were identified for the MLAs as "Address our fiscal reality" and "Do things differently."

Some at Saint Mary's saw the dangers in the arrangement but felt that they had no choice but to acquiesce. After all, the government had agreed to purchase medical services that represented one-third of the funding needed to keep the hospital open, and discussions were already occurring with private health-care providers behind the scenes as the hospital struggled for survival. The Vancouver Coastal Health Authority had already announced its intention of contracting out thousands of day surgeries and had begun talks with Saint Mary's. An agreement had been reached with the Workers' Compensation Board for rehabilitation work and the establishment of a hand clinic. Drawings had been completed for a new Downtown New Westminster Medical Clinic in the hospital building, negotiations were expected to be completed with the doctors by October and the clinic opened the following February. Other prospects included surgery and rehabilitation for the Insurance Corporation of BC (ICBC) to speed up operations and rehabilitation, developing a private eye-care clinic or obesity clinic, and even to build assisted living condos for the elderly on the hospital's parking lot. The board at Saint Mary's Hospital knew that they were facing a monumental challenge but were hopeful that they could make these deals work, and they also had the word of the health authority and provincial government that they would assist the hospital in finding other private partners to make up the funding shortfall. But they never did.

For its part, the FHA was celebrating the savings it would realize by slashing Saint Mary's operating budget. However, despite the rhetoric about preserving services, in an article in the FHA's internal newsletter they had already reported candidly that only about $5 million of the $20 million taken from the hospital's budget was intended to go into other services.[105] The rest would go to cover the deficit. Saint Mary's had been set up and deceived but hospital staff continued to work aggressively over the summer months to secure the vital funding needed from the private sector. But the concept was new and untried in British Columbia, and some private providers such as eye clinics wanted long-term assurances that, if they set up shop with Saint Mary's, the government would not flip-flop again on its promise to provide its share of funding. This was not an unreasonable position based on the hospital's treatment by the health authority and Ministry of Health over the years. The government, however, would not provide any long-term assurances.

In the early fall Saint Mary's approached the government to ask for one-time only additional funding of $15 million to allow the hospital more time to finalize its arrangements with private partners. The Fraser Health Authority still had not signed an agreement with Saint Mary's on the types of services it would purchase and the level of payment for these services. It had been hoped that it would take a month to sign this agreement, but after six months there was still no deal, although the authority had already arbitrarily cut Saint Mary's budget by two-thirds. Having failed to close the hospital in a single blow, it was slowly bleeding it to death and, despite promises of help, was doing nothing.

At the hospital, concern was increasing and Hospital Employees' Union representative Rob Newing accused the government of submitting Saint Mary's to a slow hanging on the gallows rather than a more swift and painless death. When he predicted that without more money Saint Mary's would have to shut down, the hospital was once again in the news, and once again the news was embarrassing to the FHA and a political headache for Health Minster Hansen and the provincial government. Then, when board chair Betty Wynne wrote a letter to Premier Gordon Campbell on September 19 in support of the hospital's request to have some of its funding temporarily restored on a one-time basis, events kicked into high gear. On October 1 the Premier responded that the matter had been referred to the Minister of Health. The following day Hansen appointed former provincial Auditor General George Morfitt to assess Saint Mary's business plan to determine its viability, and he was given one week to do it. He was not allowed to evaluate what success the hospital would have had if the funding had not arbitrarily been cut or if the one-time funding of $15 million had been provided, but only the probable success with the funding cuts already in place. He visited the hospital twice for a total of five hours and delivered his report to the Minister of Health on October 10. Hansen did not make the report public until November 3, giving himself more time with the report than he had given Morfitt to prepare it. The minister then delivered a copy of the report to the hospital and announced that services would be transferred out of the hospital starting immediately for reasons of "public safety." Behind the scenes the FHA had been preparing its assault and announced arrangements to transfer patients that same day. It was clear that Hansen was using the Morfitt report as justification for closing the hospital, though he would only say publicly that the report showed that the hospital's business plan was not viable—never mind that the hospital's problems were a direct result of the funding cuts of the government in the first place.

The report did say that Saint Mary's business plan was not likely to succeed, but Morfitt had actually been more specific. He said that the main problem with the plan was that it did not meet the declared financial objectives of the Fraser Health Authority, but he also said that the funding arrangement that had been concluded between the government and the hospital was feasible and should continue. His report did not recommend the closure of Saint Mary's Hospital but advised the government to consider not only finances but also its long-term objectives in health care when dealing with it. Thus the government really had three choices: close the hospital, recognize Morfitt's comment that the reduced funding for Saint Mary's was not likely to be adequate and provide temporary funding, or acknowledge its mistake and restore the hospital's funding. The government chose the most drastic option that was available. Hansen cut off all funding to Saint Mary's Hospital.

On the day Health Minister Colin Hansen announced the hospital would close, he visited Saint Mary's and met with hospital CEO Larry Odegard, board chair Betty Wynne and Sister Carla Montante. When he held a press conference at 2:30 that afternoon, as far as he was concerned, the plan to close Saint Mary's was complete. But later that day the Saint Mary's board passed a resolution that "in light of Fraser Health's decision to renege on the (without prejudice) Agreement in Principle reached in mid-April 2003, which follows their breach of the Affiliation Agreement in July 2002, the Board of Trustees of Saint Mary's Hospital has instructed its lawyers to commence legal action."[106] The motion was passed unanimously. A petition was accordingly filed in the Supreme Court on the day following the meeting. In it the board claimed that the provincial government and the Fraser Health Authority had violated numerous agreements and that the hospital had been subjected to discrimination.

What happened next came to be referred to as "the coup in the nunnery." On November 5 the Sisters announced that they would not allow the lawsuit to proceed, and shortly thereafter Sister Mary Lei Gordon emerged as the spokesperson for the Sisters of Providence and advised the hospital board that the Sisters did not wish to pursue legal action. She stated that the Sisters had been opposed to taking legal action all along. In fact, this legal option had been discussed at board meetings for months and supported by the Sisters of Providence, and the records of the meeting in which the motion was passed clearly state that the representative of the Sisters of Providence, Sister Carla Montante, was present and voted for the resolution. City councillor Casey Cook, the regular representative for the City of New Westminster on the hospital board, would later state at a city council meeting that the Sisters had a representative at the hospital board meetings for the several months during which the lawsuit was discussed and planned, and the minutes of hospital board meetings clearly stated that the Sisters had agreed for some time to take legal action as a last resort when all other options had been exhausted. What the hospital board did not know was that Sister Mary Gordon had been carrying on her own discussions with the provincial government for some time. In a simple press release, the religious order that had for so long aggressively campaigned for the hospital said: "We sincerely regret the recent events related to Saint Mary's Hospital. We are not involved in any lawsuit nor have we endorsed the initiation of legal action under our name." There was also for the first time a promise to "work with the Ministry of Health in seeking opportunities to serve the people of New Westminster in the future."[107] On November 7 Sister Gordon informed the board that she had met with Health Minister Hansen the day before and an agreement had been reached to close the hospital.

The sadness and shock at Saint Mary's was overwhelming. For nearly 117 years the Sisters of Providence had stood with the community on matters of health care. Now, in a secret meeting with the government's health minister, Saint Mary's Hospital's fate had been sealed. On November 12, hospital board chair Wynne sent letters to Health Minister Hansen, Fraser Health Authority CEO Smith and the Sisters of Providence. In her letter to Sister Gordon, Wynne asked how the board was expected to proceed with an orderly wind-down of Saint Mary's Hospital. She also asked Sister Gordon to expand on the future community role for the hospital that she and Health Minister Colin Hansen had vaguely alluded to earlier in the week. The board's quandary was due to the fact that although the Sisters of Providence owned the hospital, they did not have sole authority over its operations because the hospital's administration had been legally entrusted to a community-based board of trustees. This was a reflection of the fact that the hospital had really been a partnership between the religious order and the surrounding cities that had paid for much of its construction costs some years earlier.

Sister Mary Gordon's response was swift and shocking. Two days later she announced that "out of respect for the board," she was "releasing" its members and that a new board would be appointed immediately. The new board consisted of William Everett who was the Sisters of Providence attorney, Sister Mary Lei Gordon of the Sisters of Providence, and Ken Galbraith who was a member of the Fraser Health Authority Board. Chris Baldwin, lawyer for the Sisters, told the former board members bluntly that Minister of Health Colin Hansen had amended the hospital bylaws over the weekend to give the Sisters the power to replace them. The degree of collusion that had taken place in secret between Sister Gordon and the government was now all too clear. She announced that the new board would work with the Ministry of Health and the Fraser Health Authority to close the hospital. Her newly appointed board did not stay together for long, however. Everett resigned in January and Galbraith left the board on March 15, leaving Sister Mary Gordon and Tom Crump, a nursing home administrator and former colleague of Sister Gordon, in charge. It was rumoured that the Sister's management style was not conducive to board harmony.

Why did the Sisters of Providence take such drastic action? Explanations would be demanded from all quarters, but none were ever given. Tom Crump was appointed to oversee the closure of the hospital, but it really was the Fraser Health Authority and the provincial government, not the Sisters of Providence, that would deal with the financial and other details that needed to be resolved in the final closure of Saint Mary's Hospital. Sister Gordon announced that the Sisters essentially trusted that the government would transfer the services of Saint Mary's elsewhere. But while Sister Gordon might have been reassured, the FHA's own financial documents and letters from the Minister of Health make it clear that their reason for refusing to give in on funding Saint Mary's Hospital was that most of the money denied to Saint Mary's was going to pay down the Fraser Health Authority's deficit, which now stood at $136 million. Many would ask why Saint Mary's was the only hospital in the FHA to face such drastic measures, but the history of the hospital's shabby treatment since the creation of the health authority was answer enough. Saint Mary's, once home to orphans, was now a lone orphan itself, the last hospital with some independence and a public community board. For government and a health authority charged with cutting spending, it had been time to make this problem go away permanently.

Fighting to save Saint Mary's Hospital had been going on for so many years it had almost become part of the culture of the city and part of the routine of normal life in New Westminster, so as soon as the government announced the closure of the hospital on November 3, 2003, the Friends of Saint Mary's called an immediate meeting at the hospital. It was attended by local residents associations, the mayor and councillors from the City of New Westminster, representatives from the Council of Senior Citizens' Organizations, as well as a representative of the Catholic Archdiocese of Vancouver. From this meeting the Save Saint Mary's Hospital Coalition was born and Bill Harper was elected as its chair. A rally was planned for November 20 at Dontenwill Hall, but without the hospital actually defending itself and with the Sisters of Providence now in league with the health authority and the provincial government, all concerned knew that they faced a desperate struggle.

Coalition chair Harper opened the meeting and, ironically, was criticizing local Member of the Legislature Joyce Murray for failing to attend when she suddenly appeared. Murray maintained that she had fought to keep the hospital open but then proceeded to give the arguments for closing it. Health-care costs were rising, she said, and health care needed to be restructured. Then she reassured the audience of six hundred that there was still a future for Saint Mary's. "But I don't believe it will be as an acute-care hospital," she stated.

The booing was so loud throughout Murray's speech that little of it could be heard. "Resign!" they shouted.

"The government's decision is made," said Murray. "Everything I could do as an MLA and cabinet minister has been done,"[108] she insisted.

Near the end of the meeting an elderly nun took the microphone. "This sad occasion is my fault," she said. "I was a teacher at Saint Ann's Academy and taught Sister Mary Gordon. She was no good then and no good now. I should have expelled her," she told the gathering.

After Murray left, Dr. Irwin Stewart told the audience that the other local hospitals were already behind on their wait-lists. "Patients in this community are facing a disaster,"[109] he said. Following the rally, an editorial in the *Royal City Record* newspaper would demand to know, "Just what is Plan B? The MLA, the Fraser Health Authority, Minister of Health Services Colin Hansen, and the Sisters of Providence provide no roadmap, no plan B—in fact, nothing for anyone to actually 'get behind' . . .

Clearly the politicos, bureaucrats and Sisters want the scrambling masses to give up their fight to save the hospital as an acute-care facility."[110]

The day after Hansen announced the closure, Saint Mary's was not allowed to admit a single dying patient even though the palliative care/hospice ward had been newly refurbished just days before and specially trained staff were ready and anticipating caring for the terminally ill. No adequate replacement facility was available for months and the ward with its new home-made afghans on every bed lay vacant. Ken Coughtrey went public when Bobbie, his wife of forty-three years, had to be taken to a Burnaby care facility instead and he had to pay $850 a month for her care there. The government had promised that patients would be transferred elsewhere but had never said how

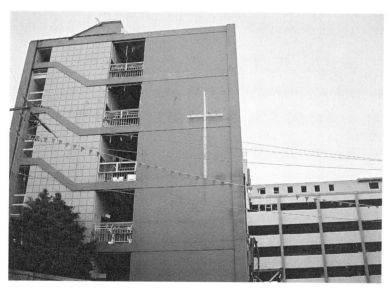

One of the first steps taken after the closure of Saint Mary's Hospital was to strip it of its religious symbols, but here the outline of a cross remains.
PHOTOGRAPH BY JAMIE McEVOY, JULY 31, 2004.

much it would cost or what that level of care that might be. Overall, the abrupt and poorly planned closure of Saint Mary's resulted in an incredible waste of resources. Following the immediate bed closures and cancellation of scheduled surgeries a full complement of highly skilled personnel were left with little to do from November 2003 until May 2004. Although a full staff reported for work daily for months, most of their hours were filled with playing cards and reading.

As Christmas approached, the coalition sponsored a Tree of Hope, which was prominently placed outside a local shopping mall. They also had three thousand lawn signs made and half of them were in place within the first week. (The situation was desperate, but the supporters of Saint Mary's had not lost their sense of humour—the sign campaign was coordinated out of a local funeral home!) In many parts of New Westminster it became impossible to walk down any street without seeing a lawn sign. Soon they began to appear throughout Burnaby and Coquitlam, hand-made signs began to pop up on lawns and in apartment windows, and a group of constituents from Health Minister Colin Hansen's riding in Vancouver put up signs there. The result was the government's worst nightmare—Saint Mary's was in the news every day for weeks.

Archbishop Adam Exner publicly backed the coalition and spoke out on behalf of the Catholic Church, making it clear that the local churches did not support the decision of the Sisters of Providence to uphold the closing of the hospital. He revealed that Health Minister Hansen had personally visited him on the day of the announcement and told him that the closure was "a done deal."[111]

As the campaign continued, city councils throughout the

region began to reassert their traditional involvement in health care that had ended with the creation of the regional health authorities. The coalition made presentations to every municipal council in the communities surrounding Saint Mary's Hospital. Peter Julian, later elected as the Member of Parliament for Burnaby–New Westminster, and Dr. Irwin Stewart led the coalition's efforts in Burnaby where the city produced its own report on the closure of the hospital. They noted that Saint Mary's served seven thousand patients a year from Burnaby. Julian, addressing the Burnaby council, described the closure of Saint Mary's as an "amputation."[112]

For a time the bureaucrats of the Fraser Health Authority attempted the same strategy, but when they actually had to function in the public eye, participate in a democratic structure and face the people's elected representatives, they were unable to win support. When Fraser Health chair Barry Forbes maintained that the pressures on Royal Columbian Hospital would decrease, a city councillor asked about the 2,700 people waiting for surgery on Saint Mary's wait-lists. Forbes responded that "doctors have wait-lists, hospitals don't have wait-lists." Burnaby city council listened for ninety minutes to the health region's CEO Smith but decided to oppose the closure of the hospital. Despite the official rhetoric that Eagle Ridge Hospital would benefit from the closure of Saint Mary's, city councils in the area of Eagle Ridge were having none of it. Port Coquitlam City Council voted five to two to oppose the closure of Saint Mary's. When FHA officials boasted the opening of two new operating rooms at Eagle Ridge, Port Coquitlam councillors were furious. The same two operating rooms had been announced in September 2003, they recalled, and had nothing to do with

Saint Mary's. (Over the next year the government announced the opening of these two operating rooms four more times.) Closing a hospital at a time when operating rooms were needed made no sense to them. (Fraser Health had the longest regional waiting lists in the province with twenty-two thousand patients in line for surgery. Ironically, with eleven thousand surgeries the previous year, Saint Mary's had handled the most surgeries in all the region's hospitals.) Councillor Arlene Crowe, commenting on the promise to deliver the services of Saint Mary's elsewhere, said, "Why the health authority wouldn't get that all up and running before is something I don't understand. It doesn't make sense to shut things down and not have an action plan."[113] And Mayor Scott Young said that he wholeheartedly supported Saint Mary's. "I think the whole problem with this is the consultation is coming after the decision."[114] In Surrey, a report ordered by city council cited lack of consultation, increasing wait-lists (more than four hundred Surrey residents were waiting for surgery at Saint Mary's), reduced access to services that were being moved far away, and the breaking up of specialized medical teams at Saint Mary's.

The mayors of New Westminster, Port Coquitlam and Burnaby, and the acting mayor of Coquitlam, held a joint news conference at Burnaby City Hall. This support by elected officials at the local level was a moral victory for Saint Mary's and it allowed for independent studies. It became clear that if the health-care system was democratic, as it had been only a few years earlier, local officials would never have agreed to close the hospital. But the system was now controlled by provincially appointed officials and powerful bureaucrats, and the locally elected officials could only join the coalition in protest.

As the coalition's work continued into January 2004, health-care horror stories continued, and a group of patients stepped forward to press their case in the media. Of particular concern was the loss of Saint Mary's breast-health clinic to patient Janet Nial, who had relied on it for the previous fifteen years. This was a highly specialized program for women who had already had cancer or were at high risk of cancer. At Saint Mary's, the time from diagnosis to treatment averaged only two weeks but, after the hospital closed, one patient who had to go elsewhere reported that it took up to two months to get results back—long enough to make the difference between life and death.

In the past Nial had also benefited from the way Saint Mary's could take pressure off Royal Columbian Hospital. In August 2000 when she had fallen and suffered a fracture, she was told in the emergency room at Royal Columbian Hospital that she would have to wait up to five days for her "emergency" operation. But a nurse had called Saint Mary's and got her a room there and she was operated on the next day. When Winifred Foster, aged 83, fell at her home on December 4, 2003, and was taken to emergency at Royal Columbian Hospital with a broken hip, she had to wait five days for an operation. Her doctor, John Albrecht, told reporters that, as had happened with Janet Nial, he used to have the option of transferring patients from the Royal Columbian emergency to Saint Mary's Hospital where they could be operated on within twenty-four hours. Albrecht said that one eighty-five-year-old man who waited for five days for hip surgery told him, "Doctor, we treat animals better than this."[115] During this same time an eight-year-old child waited three days for an operation on a broken leg at RCH.

Joe Matovic was told that he would have to wait for four years for a hip replacement and that his doctor had told him that the closure of Saint Mary's meant the wait might be longer. Matovic agreed to participate in experimental surgery so that he would get his operation sooner. But there were so many desperate patients willing to undergo the new procedure that a lottery had to be held to decide who could have the operation. Joe paid five hundred dollars for his ticket and won the lottery. The prize was a hip replacement in four months instead of four years. Independent reviews by both Burnaby and Surrey had already concluded that surgical wait-lists were likely to be impacted by the closure of Saint Mary's, despite the reassurance of the government.

Meanwhile, the fire department had inspected Royal Columbian Hospital and threatened action because the emergency department was so overcrowded that it posed a safety hazard. So many patients were lying on stretchers in the hallways waiting for emergency treatment or a hospital bed that the exits were blocked. This was exactly what Dr. Irwin Stewart, a veteran of the fight for Saint Mary's going back to the days of Health Minister Rafe Mair in the 1980s, had predicted the previous November—that by transferring one-third of Saint Mary's patients to the Royal Columbian, patients "will lie in stretchers in the hallway of emergency."[116]

The media attention to patients' horror stories was widespread and damaging to the claims from the government that all was well. The Fraser Health Authority responded with an expensive ad campaign but it contained few specifics and the horror stories continued. In February—but only after it was publicly revealed by the coalition—the FHA admitted that it did not know how it would deal with the 1,200 people who were waiting for cataract surgery at Saint Mary's. It seems the health authority had somehow expected a thousand fewer people to have operations in the region the year after Saint Mary's closed.

On February 4 Fraser Health CEO Bob Smith agreed to give a ninety-minute interview to the *Royal City Record*. Commenting on the amalgamation of the health regions, Smith said candidly, "These changes cause an emasculation of the people who work here," and then added, "There aren't very many successful mergers of that size." He said that health care was no longer a place to plan on having a job for life: "To count on us for that for the future is not on . . . The traditional trust—I can't offer that. It's not part of a sustainable health-care system."[117] When Smith mentioned that the region would need another hospital in ten to fifteen years, reporter Lori Pappajohn asked him if it wasn't shortsighted to be closing Saint Mary's only to build another hospital later. Smith responded vaguely with "Saint Mary's closing—that's a good point."[118] (Just a year after giving this interview Smith was mired in a fresh controversy. He had sent an email to staff at Surrey Memorial telling the administration there to deal with emergency-room overcrowding by discharging patients more quickly. He was fired by his boss, Barry Forbes; perhaps Smith had become a bit too candid for the government's liking.)

Three months after announcing the closure of Saint Mary's the Fraser Health Authority finally agreed to hold a public meeting to discuss it. That meeting was held at the Metrotown Hilton in Burnaby and was a public relations fiasco for the health authority. Over three hundred Saint Mary's supporters crowded into a small hotel ballroom to listen to Barry Forbes and Bob Smith attempt to justify the hospital's closure. Fraser Health security guards sealed off the area as the room became full and physically barred access to many who wished to attend the meeting. When several persons objected to the dark-clad security guards spread throughout the room like a scene from a Hollywood movie, the audience was told by the head of "issues management" for the authority, Helen Carkner, that extra security was now a standard precaution at health authority board meetings. In fact, the Fraser Health Authority and its department of Issues Management had hired its own Director of Protection Services.

The Save Saint Mary's Hospital Coalition called for a public inquiry into the Fraser Health Authority and the call was quickly supported by New Westminster and Burnaby city councils. The government rejected the idea immediately but the press was very interested in the questions the public was asking. Why had the health authority not assisted Saint Mary's to secure private funding after they had promised to do so? Why had the health authority stalled for months, refusing to sign a funding agreement? Did the government make any promises to cover liabilities in return for the Sisters of Providence toeing the line? Why was Saint Mary's singled out for the cuts? How was the $20 million that was going to be saved every year from closing Saint Mary's to be spent? What impact would this have on health care? Would the government agree that the estimated $15 million they were spending on severance packages for Saint Mary's staff was an unnecessary waste of resources? (Ironically this was exactly the amount Saint Mary's needed to stay open.)

The coalition was raising issues that would have had their day in court had Health Minister Hansen not rewritten the hospital bylaws to allow for the board to be fired. Why was the government preventing the issue from getting into the courts? The coalition believed, as did the lawyers who had worked for the old Saint Mary's board, that the Fraser Health Authority had acted illegally when it first moved to cut the hospital's funding back in June 2002 without consultation with the hospital's board, and that the hospital board had been forced to agree to dramatic cuts to its budget under duress, without the protection of the provincial agreement with religious hospitals being upheld by the government. Coalition chair Harper told Forbes and Smith, "You can shut the door and turn the lock, but we're not going away."[119]

At the end of February, MLA Joyce Murray hosted Premier Gordon Campbell for a private gathering in her home and, as he arrived, Campbell could not have avoided seeing the sea of "Save Saint Mary's" on the neighbours' lawns. Long-time Saint Mary's advocate Paul Levy, also a guest at this gathering, took the opportunity to question the premier. "If there are no good reasons for closing the hospital," Levy told him, "then there has to be a bad one."[120] Campbell appeared to be angry about the confrontation and, after giving a speech at a local event, quickly left town.

It was now generally accepted that the hospital was closing, but since the official closure date was not until later that May, the coalition commissioned a poll of residents in New Westminster, North Surrey, Coquitlam and South Burnaby, to be conducted by the Mustel Group. The results were overwhelmingly in favour of the Save Saint Mary's Coalition and against the government. In fact, 95 percent of those who expressed an opinion were opposed to closing the hospital. But if the coalition had hoped that the poll results would make the government more pragmatic and open to dialogue, they were about to be sadly disappointed.

Meanwhile, Saint Mary's CEO Larry Odegard and Vice-President of Finance Steve Loader had been relieved of their duties at the hospital and sent home on full pay. A few days later Karl Crosby, Director of Public Relations and Development, was summarily fired from his position as hospital spokesperson on the vague charge that he had breached hospital confidentiality by advising Saint Mary's Foundation board members of the removal of Odegard and Loader. But the same press release that announced the suspensions of the hospital's administrators also announced an investigation into the hospital's finances, casting a cloud of suspicion over senior managers who had done absolutely nothing wrong. "This was absurd and petty," said Crosby. "The removal of Odegard and Loader and the impending financial review was public knowledge within the hospital and in the community." However, it was clear that the new administration was getting rid of anyone they thought might be opposed to the closure of the hospital—first the board of trustees and then the hospital's senior management.

The event that had actually sparked the health authority's decision to hold a financial review had occurred on the other side of the country. Hal Schmidt, the former head of Saint Mary's who had defended the hospital so ably against the Hay Report and the health authority's attempts to close the hospital in 1998, had been dismissed from a hospital in Halifax where he had recently been appointed CEO after someone associated with the closure of Saint Mary's had informed the hospital board there that Schmidt did not hold the accounting degree that he had claimed on his resumé. Although he was clearly well qualified for the position and had completed all the necessary requirements as a chartered accountant, he had not written the final examination.

No details of the FHA's financial review were ever made public, but a press release announced that the audit had been turned over to the RCMP for criminal investigation. This was not actually true at that time. The report had not been turned over to anybody, but when the coalition and the media discovered there was no investigation underway, the FHA did make an attempt to give the report to the RCMP. They refused to become involved. The coalition then called for the audit to be made public. "If the government is going to selectively release some information related to a scandal, it should open up the whole issue to a public and independent process,"[121] said coalition organizer Jaimie McEvoy.

Meanwhile, the new administration set up to oversee the hospital's closure continued to express shock, betrayal and disappointment over the "wrong-doing," but they would never explain what was behind their vindictive and damning claims. In fact, the report's actual contents were kept so secret that not even the hospital's Vice-President of Finance, Stephen Loader, was able to obtain a copy. Then in March, Loader, a twenty-year employee of the hospital with an impeccable work record, was fired with no explanation. Why those closing Saint Mary's Hospital would purposely attack first Schmidt and then other senior administrators of the hospital was unclear, but it may have been to deflect public criticism of the government and the health authority by suggesting wrongdoing at the hospital. Whatever their object may have been, it soon became very clear that the financial review, the attack on former CEO Schmidt and the firings of Loader and Crosby were vindictive and punitive without cause or justification.

Finally, the report, having been rejected by the RCMP, was then taken to the New Westminster police. They also rejected it. Staff Sergeant Derek Dickson of the New Westminster police services would later say, "We're quite comfortable nothing of a criminal nature was revealed in the report. We are quite happy to wash our hands of it."[122] Unfortunately, the FHA press releases had already been issued, and the damage had been done. Former board chair Betty Wynne told the *Royal City Record* that a forensic audit of the hospital's finances had been "totally unnecessary" as all financial records and yearly audits performed by major accounting firms were impeccable. She speculated that "there was vindictiveness behind the actions of those responsible,"[123] and city councillor Casey Cook called the entire matter "nothing more than a PR stunt."[124]

Sister Mary Gordon, who had been so quick to go public with her accusations, would not go public with her acceptance of the findings of the police report. But Tom Crump, who was in charge of closing the hospital, announced that the report, having been rejected after unsuccessful attempts to interest the RCMP and the New Westminster police, would now be shopped around to "other agencies."[125] And the Fraser Health Authority then attempted to punish Schmidt on their own accord by publicly announcing that the authority was suing him, a threat they never pursued.

The final blow for Saint Mary's Hospital came in the

summer of 2004 when it was announced that the Sisters of Providence had sold the hospital to Bosa Developments for $4.1 million, a bargain basement price considering the property had been recently assessed at $7.3 million.

Behind the scenes the Catholic Archdiocese of Vancouver had been fighting this sale for months because they were committed to continuing the mission of compassionate care to which Saint Mary's had been dedicated. The Sisters' response had been to say that if the Archdiocese wanted to buy it they could; unfortunately, the Archdiocese did not have that kind of money. When the hospital's funding was cut, Archbishop Exner had asked Premier Campbell to personally intervene but nothing came of it, so the Archbishop's Vicar of Health, Reverend Bernard Rossi, had then set out to assist Saint Mary's in its attempts to find alternative funding for the hospital. Thus, when Health Minister Hansen insisted that the hospital's closure was a done deal, the Archdiocese of Vancouver had immediately sought a meeting with the Sisters of Providence to find common ground on the issue. That meeting had not taken place until November 28, almost a full month after the withdrawal of the lawsuit and the firing of the hospital board.

On December 5 Sister Carla Montante, the president of the order in western Canada, sent a letter to the Archbishop informing him that the hospital board was fired for having failed to follow the Sisters' instructions and that, "their disregard for our wishes left us no choice." She made no mention of the fact that she had actually sat in on the meetings where the lawsuit was discussed and had voted with the hospital board to proceed with legal action, or that the Minister of Health had rewritten the hospital bylaws so that the board could be removed. But her letter also revealed another motivation for the Sisters' actions, one that was never made public and that came directly from the provincial government: "Had the Minister exercised his authority under the Health Act to dismiss the board and the administrator and appointed a public administrator, we would have lost our assets." The letter also says that delaying lay-off notices in an attempt to fight the closing of the hospital would have exposed the Sisters to possible liabilities that they could not afford. (According to Vicar of Health Rossi, the Sisters had been advised by the government that they would be liable for the expenditures of the hospital.) Sister Montante's letter goes on to say: "Saint Mary's was our first mission in western Canada and we have not lost sight of that. This is a time of grief and loss for us all. As we rely on our Provident God for wisdom and strength, please pray for us and for a future role for Saint Mary's. We have not given up on faith-based care and we are working to find a way to preserve its presence in New Westminster."[126] The Sisters of Providence would come to find, as had the hospital board before them, that attempting to negotiate with the Fraser Health Authority was pointless.

As it became clear that the hospital was going to close, the Archbishop and Monsignor Rossi decided to take the necessary steps to block any sale of the hospital. The Sisters would then be required to allow the hospital building to continue being used by the Archdiocese or some other group for the mission for which it was built—providing compassionate health care to people of all faiths. There was also the possibility that, if the Sisters wished to do so, the hospital could be donated to an organization like the Archdiocese or to Providence Health Care.

While this was going on behind the scenes, a committee in

New Westminster headed by Paul Levy and Michael Crean was still hoping that the building might have a future use for the common good of the community. Low-rental housing for the disabled, shelter for the homeless and low-rental or even free space for non-profit groups were all concepts that were being explored in an attempt to duplicate what had happened when Saint Vincent's Hospital in Vancouver had recently been closed and demolished. That hospital's programs had all been kept within Providence Health and the land had been used to build a new facility for the elderly. However, when Hal Schmidt had suggested that option earlier, the Archdiocese had written to the Sisters in pursuit of a similar arrangement, but nothing had come of it.

But now the Archdiocese was confident that any sale of the hospital not related to the hospital's mission would be blocked by the Vatican, and that a group like the one headed by Levy and Crean might be able to approach the Sisters and make an offer. The Archdiocese was counting on the fact that, under canonical law, any sale of land over a certain value requires the Vatican's approval and the sale price has to be based on the actual value of the property. In Canada the limit before permission is required is $4.3 million. This rule was intended to prevent a religious order from selling property in which the community at large had a vested interest, as was clearly the case with Saint Mary's Hospital.

Although the Sisters' intention to sell had not been made public, on March 20, 2004, Archbishop Roussin wrote to Rome advising that the Sisters were planning to sell the hospital, apparently without the required permission. The Vatican reassured the Archbishop that his assent would be sought should any such request by the Sisters to sell the hospital be made to Rome. The Archdiocese therefore thought that it had effectively blocked any possible sale and that, although Saint Mary's would not be used as a hospital, it had once again been saved. Thus, when the sale to Bosa Development Corporation for $4.1 million was announced less than a month later, the reaction of Monsignor Rossi and colleagues was one of shock. How could it be? The assessed value of the city-block-sized property was $7.3 million and the cost to replace the nine-storey building would far exceed this figure. Of course, it was no accident that the Sisters of Providence sold the property for $4.1 million. They had not advertised to attract the best price or invited proposals for the future use of the site. Instead, they had quietly found a buyer who would pay just below the threshold of $4.3 million that would have required Vatican approval.

Thus, despite the requirements of canonical law, Rome knew nothing about the sale. In a letter of April 29, 2004, Piergiorgio Silvano Nesti of the Vatican confirmed that the Sisters of Providence had not requested approval. They had simply gone ahead and done it. Nesti assured the Archbishop that had Rome been asked for permission as required, Exner would have been asked for his approval. "It is the practice of this Dicastery to ask the assent of the Bishop of the place before conceding the canonical permission," he wrote.[127]

The hopes of the local Catholic Church and the Save Saint Mary's Coalition to make compassionate use of the now empty hospital building had been finally and irrevocably dashed. When a letter was sent from Rome asking the Sisters about the sale, they responded that they thought that they had acted in

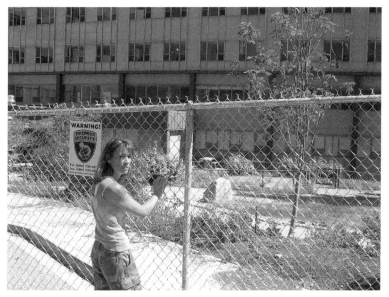

Katherine Gordon was one of the thousands born at Saint Mary's Hospital because her strongly Protestant mother chose it for her birth. "Mom said that she had been a patient there and everyone had been so kind. She really felt that they were extraordinary." PHOTOGRAPH BY JAIMIE McEVOY, JULY 31, 2004.

good faith and that their selling price was below the threshold, even though selling below value was exactly the kind of action that the rule was intended to prevent. For its part, Rome accepted the Sisters' explanation and informed the Archbishop that the matter would be dropped, but Monsignor Rossi still strongly objected to the sale. "But what could we do?" he said when interviewed later. "Church law had been broken, but it's not like we have police or courts to enforce the law . . . I'm sorry to say it, but there was subterfuge. I mean, why let us know of the sale through the newspapers?" Then he added, "Many Sisters worked there and worked for nothing, but they didn't do that alone. The land was donated, and the hospital was built and supported by the whole community."[128] He was not, of course, the only one to question whether the Sisters of Charity of Providence were legally entitled to the millions they received as a result of the sale.

In one final twist Sister Mary Gordon wrote to New Westminster City Council in support of the demolition of Saint Mary's Hospital.

Epilogue

Revisit to Health Care

AS SAINT MARY'S HOSPITAL was being demolished during the summer of 2005, I occasionally visited the site. As the wrecking ball shattered the walls, passersby would pause and watch for a few minutes as the 117-year old Catholic mission of "compassionate care to people of all faiths" came to an end. During my visits, there was also a small but steady stream of people quietly making their way to the site, usually alone, and it seemed as if they were making a pilgrimage to a holy place. Often they were crying. I spoke to several of them. Many had been born at Saint Mary's Hospital and others had their lives improved by the care they had received there over the years. But what they all had in common was a memory of the very special care they had received.

That summer as Saint Mary's Hospital was reduced to rubble, I was taken to Royal Columbia Hospital by ambulance. It was my personal opportunity to experience the present health-care system for real. The ambulance attendants told me that it was too bad that I was not well enough to go to a clinic as I could expect to wait several hours in emergency before being treated. How right they were. I waited four hours for an electrocardiogram. It was another six hours before an exhausted physician, visibly stressed, his hands shaking, was able to examine me. I was told that if the pains persisted to come back tomorrow. Throughout the long wait and a shift change, the ambulance attendants sat with me, unable to leave me until I had been checked in by the hospital. Next to me, an elderly woman, who had been found lying on her balcony in a rainstorm, was given basic first aid for hypothermia by ambulance attendants, but hours passed before she received any medical attention. I watched as the emergency department lost track of patients, as stretchers of seriously ill and injured patients lined the walls and a handful of overworked nurses and doctors struggled to handle the most urgent cases. It was chaos and brought to mind the kind of scene one might expect to see on television during a major disaster, and I couldn't help thinking that there was a time not long ago when Saint Mary's had been the release valve for the Royal Columbian's emergency room.

As I researched and wrote this book, the newspapers were full of stories about the state of emergency rooms in British Columbia hospitals. A headline in *The Vancouver Sun* read: "Overcrowded ER Killing Patients at Royal Columbian Report Says." And in the article that followed Dr. Sheldon Glazier was quoted as saying, "People have been dying waiting on ambulance stretchers in our emergency room and here is a document that actually confirms it." Staff at Burnaby Hospital have said they need more emergency room space as patient visits are up from forty-five thousand to forty-nine thousand in just four years. The Fraser Health Authority blamed the increase on a spate of winter flu cases.

There is a tendency for health officials to reassure themselves that the problems of health care in Canada are the same all over the world. My research indicates that most are doing better than we are. So much good might have been done with the Saint Mary's Hospital building and grounds. In my neighbourhood, the Hospitality Project at Shiloh-Sixth Avenue United Church has stepped forward to establish a clothing exchange and provide a cup of coffee, a place to sit, and support to the Food Bank, the largest in the Lower Mainland. A few blocks in the other direction, the Purpose Society has been operating an alternative school and other programs for troubled youth and street kids for several years. Fraserside, which started as a clothing exchange, has become one of the largest service organizations in the region. Just down the street is Family Place, providing parenting programs and other support for parents of young children. Down the hill from Saint Mary's is the Cliff Block where the Lookout Society has converted one of the most crime-ridden and desperately poor buildings in the city into a fully renovated and staffed shelter, providing a place to live and education for homeless people, some of whom have not had shelter in many years. Within walking distance, Olivet Baptist Church, Queens Avenue United Church, Sixth Avenue United Church, Saint Aidan's Presbyterian Church and Saint Barnabas Anglican Church all continue the tradition of providing compassionate services for the good of the whole community. And to its credit, the Saint Mary's Hospital Foundation, now working as the Saint Mary's Health Foundation, refused to shut down when the hospital closed. Since 2004 it has continued to support the greatest need and donated over $500,000 to local health care.

The need for an improved health-care system has never been greater. Perhaps elected politicians will insist on the return of democracy to the health-care system and restore the role that local communities once played in their own well-being. Perhaps then, letters to the government, petitions bearing thousands of signatures, attendance at public meetings, lawn signs, and direct personal appeals to elected representatives will stand a greater chance of getting a fair hearing on such a vital issue as health care.

Acknowledgements

THIS BOOK WOULD NOT HAVE BEEN POSSIBLE without the gracious support of many others. Thanks must especially go to the Saint Mary's Health Foundation for extensive support and commitment to the memory of Saint Mary's Hospital. Particular thanks to Paul Levy, Betty Wynne, Dr. Irwin Stewart, Bernie Bilodeau and Bev Welsh, all of whom provided valuable information, feedback and necessary proofreading. Particular thanks go to Karl Crosby, who served as editor of my initial manuscript. Special thanks also to Betty Keller, who served as the editor of my final manuscript.

I want to give very important recognition to those who provided invaluable personal support. My partner Stacy Ashton, who acted as research assistant, confidante and advisor, and who was graciously supportive and patient with the many late nights of work. Thanks to my long-time friend Katherine Gordon, who first encouraged me to write and publish and who made it possible. Thanks to my dear friend Melanie Mora for the inspiration to believe in the good. Special thanks to my very dear family: my Dad Dave, Mom Rose, David, Tammy, Colleen and Martin, and all the grandparents, aunts, uncles, grand-uncles and grand-aunts, cousins and second cousins who taught a little boy the value of love and community, and to my many friends for their support and patience as I completed this book.

Archie Miller, Gavin Hainsworth, Katherine Freund-Hainsworth and Jim Wolf, all authors of history in their own right, provided knowledgeable feedback and information on historical material. Mary Tews, Anne Kroeker and Irene Petruk provided valuable information on the hospital's auxiliary. Thanks to Margaret Hickey for her information on the Local Council of Women.

I am indebted to several archives and libraries, particularly the staff of the New Westminster Public Library, the New Westminster Museum and Archives, the British Columbia Archives and the Saint Paul's Hospital Archives, each of whose staff and volunteers provided me with many hours of kind assistance. Others include the National Library and Archives of Canada, Library of Congress, Vancouver Public Library, City of Vancouver Archives, Burnaby Public Library, Richmond Museum, Glenbow Archives (Alberta), McGill University Archives, Spartanburg Technical College Library, City of Surrey Archives, Mission Museum, Providence Archives (Seattle), City of Coquitlam Archives, Vancouver Museum, University of British Columbia Library and Archives, McCord Museum and the Legislative Library of British Columbia, all of whom provided information and assistance.

Thanks also to the *Royal City Record*, and especially to Gary E. Slavin (Slavin Creative Design), who took on the daunting task of photography work and the initial design work, and to Gianni Dente, who kindly assisted. Special thanks also to Kate O'Hara, Patricia Wolfe and Arbutus Books. There were many others who are too numerous to mention, and some of whom would prefer to remain anonymous. To all of you, many thanks. A special thank you to those Sisters of Providence who kept the faith, kept the home fires burning in the very heart of our community, and helped our town and our province build its traditions of tolerance and compassion. And, finally, to the people of New Westminster, the little city that I love, and whose civic spirit, pride in history, and traditions in support of the common good are second to none.

—Jaimie McEvoy

Recommended Reading

Adams, George Worthington. *Doctors in Blue: The Medical History of the Union Army in the Civil War.* Louisiana State University Press, Baton Rouge, 1952, 1980.

Brown, Debra J. *The Challenge of Caring: A History of Women and Health Care in British Columbia.* Ministry of Health, Victoria. 2000.

Campbell Hurd-Mead M.D., Kate. *A History of Women in Medicine.* Haddam Press, Haddam, Connecticut. 1938.

Freud-Hainsworth, Katherine and Gavin Hainsworth. *A New Westminster Album.* Dundurn Press, Toronto, 2005.

Glavin, Terry. *Amongst God's Own: The Enduring Legacy of Saint Mary's Mission.* Longhouse Publishing, Mission, 2002.

Harrison, Eunice M.L. *The Judge's Wife: Memoirs of a British Columbia Pioneer.* Ronsdale Press, Vancouver, 2002.

Leonoff, Cyril Edel. *Pioneers, Pedlars and Prayer Shawls: The Jewish Communities in British Columbia and the Yukon.* Sono Nis Press, Victoria, 1978.

Luxton, Donald (ed.). *Building the West: The Early Architects of British Columbia.* Talon Books. Vancouver. 2003.

Maher, Sister Mary Denis. *To Bind Up the Wounds: Catholic Sister Nurses in the U.S. Civil War.* Louisiana State University Press, Baton Rouge, 1989.

Miller, Archie and Dale Kerr. *The Great Fire of 1898.* A Sense of History Research Services Inc., New Westminster, 1998.

O'Keefe, Betty and Ian MacDonald. *Dr. Fred and the Spanish Lady: Fighting the Killer Flu.* Heritage House, Surrey, BC. 2004.

Pullem, Hellen C. *New Westminster: The Real Story Of How It All Began.* Hawkscourt Group, New Westminster, 1985.

Rogers, Fred. *Shipwrecks of British Columbia.* Douglas and McIntyre, Vancouver, 1973, 1980.

Sanford, Barrie. *Royal Metal: The People, Times and Trains of New Westminster Bridge.* National Railway Historical Society, British Columbia chapter, Vancouver, 2004.

The Little Medical Guide of the Sisters of Charity of Providence. Sisters of Charity of Providence, Montreal. 1889.

The Statue of Mother Joseph, A Sister of Providence. United States Congress. United States Government Printing Office. Washington, D.C. 1980.

Tolmie, William Fraser. *Journals 1830–1843.* Mitchell Press, Vancouver, 1963.

Wolf, Jim. *Royal City: A Photographic History of New Westminster, 1858–1960.* Heritage House, surrey, BC, 2005.

Woodland, Alan. *New Westminster: The Early Years, 1858–1898.* Nunaga Publishing Company, New Westminster, 1973.

Notes

1. Harrison, Eunice M.L., *The Judge's Wife: Memoirs of a British Columbia Pioneer* (Ronsdale Press, Vancouver, 2002) 22–24.

2. Harrison, 22–24.

3. Pullem, Hellen C., *New Westminster: The Real Story of How It All Began* (Hawkscourt Group, New Westminster, 1985) 100.

4. Hill, Beth, *Sappers: The Royal Engineers in British Columbia* (Horsdal & Schubart, Ganges, BC, 1987) 91.

5. Adolph, Val, *In the Context of its Time: A History of Woodlands* (Government of British Columbia, Ministry of Social Sevices, Richmond, 1996).

6. Elliott, Gordon R., *Barkerville, Quesnel & the Cariboo Gold Rush* (Douglas & McIntyre, Vancouver, 1978) 75.

7. Adolph, Val.

8. Elliott, Gordon R. *Barkerville, Quesnel & the Cariboo Gold Rush* (Douglas & McIntyre, Vancouver, 1978) 75.

9. *Letters of Reverend Fouquet, OMI, June 8, 1863*, (Mission de la Congregation de Missionaire Oblates de Marie Immacule [OMI Mission] III) 197.

10. D'Herbomez, Louis-Joseph, OMI, Letter to Sister Praxedes, October 30, 1875.

11. D'Herbomez, Letter.

12. D'Herbomez, Letter.

13. Mother Amable, Sisters of Providence, Letter to Sister Joseph of the Sacred Heart. May 15, 1886.

14. *Deliberations of the Corporation of the Sisters of Charity of the House of Providence*, 31–32.

15. *Deliberations.*

16. "The New Hospital," *The Mainland Guardian*, July 21, 1886, 3.

17. Quesnelle, S.P., Hortense, "Precis of Chronicles of St. Mary's Hospital, New Westminster, BC" (unpublished, circa 1978) 1.

18. "At the Recent Fire at the Arlington," *The Mainland Guardian*, January 19, 1887, 2.

19. "At the Recent Fire at the Arlington."

20. Ellis, Lucia, *Cornerstone: The Story of St. Vincent's, Oregon's First Permanent Hospital, Its Formative Years,* (St. Vincent Medical Foundation, Portland, Oregon, 1975) 22. As cited in Clevenger, Sydney, "St. Vincent's and the Sisters of Providence: Oregon's First Permanent Hospital," *Oregon Historical Quarterly*, Portland, Oregon. Summer 2001, Vol. 10, No. 2.

21. *Statue of Mother Joseph, A Sister of Providence* (United States Congress, United States Government Printing Office, Washington, D.C. 1980) 60.

22. *Statue of Mother Joseph.*

23. *Statue of Mother Joseph*, 5.

24. *Statue of Mother Joseph*, 54.

25. *Statue of Mother Joseph*, 6.

26. *Statue of Mother Joseph.*

27. As cited in *Statue of Mother Joseph*, 8. Original source information not given.

28. BC Archives A-02133 and BC Medical Association Archives.

29. Commager, H.S. ed.. *The Blue and the Gray: The Story of the Civil War As Told by Participants* (Indianapolis and New York, 1950, II) 769–795.

30. *The Journals of William Fraser Tolmie, Physician and Pioneer.* (Mitchell Press, Vancouver, 1963).

31. Quesnelle, S.P., Hortense, "Precis of Chronicles of St. Mary's Hospital, New Westminster, BC" (unpublished, circa 1978) 3.

32. "Reminiscences of Seventy-Two Years: St. Mary's Hospital, New Westminster, BC." (author and original publication information unknown, circa 1958).

33. Quesnelle, 3.

34. "Reminiscences."

35. Quesnelle, 3.

36. Letter, New Westminster Local Council of Women, October 14, 1898 (New Westminster Museum and Archives).

37. Quesnelle, 4.

38. Quesnelle, 4.

39. Patient register, 1887–1907 (Manuscript #302, New Westminster Museum and Archives).

40. Receipts, October 1898 (Manuscript #302, New Westminster Museum and Archives).

41. Rogers, Fred, *Shipwrecks of British Columbia* (Douglas & McIntyre, Vancouver, 1973, 1980) 209.

42. Quesnelle, 6.

43. Quesnelle, 7.

44. Quesnelle, 7.

45. Quesnelle, 7.

46. O'Keefe, Betty, and Ian McDonald, *Dr. Fred and the Spanish Lady: Fighting the Killer Flu* (Heritage House, Surrey, BC, 2004) 136.

47. Quesnelle, S.P., Hortense, "Precis of Chronicles of St. Mary's Hospital, New Westminster, BC" (unpublished, circa 1978).

48. "Hollyweird North," *Western Living Magazine*, December 2001.

49. By-laws of the St. Mary's Hospital Auxiliary, 1947.

50. Minutes, St. Mary's Hospital Auxiliary, June 15, 1948.

51. Minutes, St. Mary's Hospital Auxiliary, May 1, 1947.

52. Quesnelle, 17.

53. Quesnelle, 19.

54. Quesnelle, 25.

55. Quesnelle, 26.

56. Quesnelle, 28.

57. Quesnelle, 29.

58. Quesnelle, 31.

59. Quesnelle, 32.

60. Quesnelle, 32.

61. Quesnelle, 33.

62. "Council opposes hospital downgrading," *The Columbian*, July 8, 1980.

63. *The Columbian*, July 8, 1980.

64. "Changes in St. Mary's 'stupid,'" *The Columbian*, July 10, 1980.

65. *The Columbian*, July 10, 1980.

66. Interview with Rafe Mair, July 22, 2005.

67. Interview, July 22, 2005.

68. Interview, July 22, 2005.

69. "St. Mary's directors may appeal directly to Mair," *The Columbian*, July 17, 1980.

70. *The Columbian*, July 17, 1980.

71. "Hospital decision will kill Socreds," *The Columbian*, August 8, 1980.

72. Interview with Rafe Mair, July 22, 2005.

73. Smith, Lorne, "Fight over St. Mary's lost at GVRD," *The Columbian*, November 27, 1980.

74. Smith, Lorne.

75. Interview, July 22, 2005.

76. Interview, July 22, 2005.

77. "It's not how we're changing . . . It's why," Pamphlet, Simon Fraser Health Region, 1998.

78. Interview with Hal Schmidt, September 23, 2005.

79. Schmidt.

80. "Sisters of Providence opposed to Acute Care Recommendations," Press release, St. Mary's Hospital, September 14, 1998.

81. Press release.

82. Hilborn, Dan, "Doctors Oppose Hay Group Health Plans," *The Record*, October 11, 1998.

83. "Friends of St. Mary's Hospital," Pamphlet.

84. Pappajohn, Lori, "15,000-Name Petition Opposes Health Plan," *The Record*, October 25, 1998.

85. Chow, Wanda, "St. Mary's Supporters Gear Up for Protest," *New Westminster News Leader*, September 23, 1998.

86. Pappajohn, Lori, "Crowds expected to pack library at tonight's health meeting," *The Record*, September 23, 1998.

87. "Meeting raises serious doubts," Editorial, *The Record*, September 27, 1998.

88. Chow, Wanda, "St. Mary's draws support," *New Westminster News Leader,* September 27, 1998.

89. Pappajohn, Lori, "Protesters pack meeting to oppose plans to radically alter St. Mary's," *The Record,* September 27, 1998.

90. Pappajohn, Lori, "1,200 people turn out in support of St. Mary's," *The Record,* October 4, 1998. 1.

91. Pappajohn, 3.

92. Hilborn, Dan, "Protests could kill report on health care," *The Record,* December 6, 1998, 3.

93. Hilborn, 3.

94. "Remarks from Dennis Cocke, Board Chair, Simon Fraser Health Region," A Joint Press Conference on the Agreement between the Simon Fraser Health Region Board and the St. Mary's Hospital Board, January 8, 1999.

95. "Remarks."

96. Michalski, John. Letter from St. Mary's Hospital chair to Simon Fraser Health Region chair Paul McDonnell, April 20, 2000.

97. Smyth, Michael, "Fight over St. Mary's Hospital does bring back some memories," *The Province.*

98. Pappajohn, Lori, "New boards responsible for 'businesslike' operations," *The Record,* 7.

99. Interview with Hal Schmidt, September 25, 2005.

100. Schmidt.

101. "1,200 people rally against plan to shut 'model' hospital," *The Province,* September 20, 2002.

102. Harrison, Don, "St. Mary's Hospital wins reprieve from review panel," *The Province,* January 8, 2003.

103. McLellan, Julie, "St. Mary's gets a new deal," *The Record,* April 16, 2003.

104. "Beloved New West Hosptial survives with new role," *The Vancouver Sun,* April 16, 2003, B2.

105. *InFocus,* August 5, 2003.

106. Minutes, St. Mary's Hospital Board of Trustees, Meeting in Camera, November 3, 2003, 1600 hours.

107. Press release by the Sisters of Providence of British Columbia, November 5, 2003.

108. Turnau, Amber, "'Resign' rally-goers chant at MLA," *The Record*, November 22, 2003, 8.

109. Turnau.

110. "Just what is Plan B?" Editorial, *The Record*, November 22, 2003, 6.

111. Turnau, Amber, "Archbishop backs Coalition," *The Record*, November 29, 2003, 8.

112. Lau, Alfie, "Burnaby backs St. Mary's Fight," *The Record*, November 26, 2003, 4.

113. Blains, Simone, "Put PoCo's name on the list to save St. Mary's Hospital," *Coquitlam Now*, December 10, 2003, 3.

114. Blains.

115. Pappajohn, Lori, "Elderly woman waits five days for RCH surgery," *The Record*, January 24, 2004, 4.

116. Turnau, Amber, "'Resign,' rally-goers chant at MLA," *The Record*, November 22, 2003, 1.

117. Hilborn, Dan, "Health boss speaks out," *The Record*, February 4, 2004, 3.

118. Pappajohn, Lori, "Waiting lists a constant challenge," *The Record*, February 4, 2004, 3.

119. Weir, David, "St. Mary's group calls for public inquiry," *News Leader*, February 7, 2004, 10.

120. Pappajohn, Lori, "Premier gets an earful," *The Record*, February 28, 2004, 3.

121. Pappajohn, Lori, "RCMP says audit a city police issue," *The Record*, March 17, 2004.

122. Lau, Alfie, "St. Mary's case was unfounded," *The Record*, April 28, 2004, 1.

123. Lau.

124. Lau.

125. Weir, David, "St. Mary's books still under review," *News Leader*, May 5, 2004, 11.

126. Montante, Sister Carla, S.P. Letter to Most Reverend Adam Exner, OMI, December 5, 2003.

127. Nesti, Piergiorgio Silvano, Letter to Archbishop Raymond Roussin, April 29, 2004.

128. Interview with Reverend Bernard Rossi, August 26, 2005.

Index